THE
EVERYTHING

HERBAL REMEDIES
BOOK

Feel better naturally using simple treatments
and home remedies

M.J. Abadie

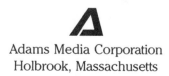

Adams Media Corporation
Holbrook, Massachusetts

An Everything Series Book.
"Everything" is a trademark of Adams Media Corporation.

Published by Adams Media Corporation
260 Center Street, Holbrook, MA 02343. U.S.A.
www.adamsmedia.com

ISBN: 1-58062-331-X

Printed in the United States of America.

J I H G F E D C B A

Library of Congress Cataloging-in-Publication Data
Abadie, M. J.
The everything herbal remedies book / M. J. Abadie.–1st ed.
p.   cm.
ISBN 1-58062-331-X
1. Herbs–Therapeutic use. 2. Medicinal plants. I. Title.
RM666.H33 A174   2000
615'.321–dc21   -029292
CIP

This publication is designed to provide accurate and authoritative information with regard to the subject matter covered. It is sold with the understanding that the publisher is not engaged in rendering legal, accounting, or other professional advice. If legal advice or other expert assistance is required, the services of a competent professional person should be sought.
— From a *Declaration of Principles* jointly adopted by a Committee of the American Bar Association and a Committee of Publishers and Associations

Illustrations by Barry Littmann and Kathie Kelleher

This book is available at quantity discounts for bulk purchases.
For information, call 1-800-872-5627.

To Susan Shaw

My dear friend and herbal "walking encyclopedia," with gratitude
for sharing her extensive knowledge of herbs and their many
uses—and for an enduring friendship.

Contents

Part One
Historical Use of Herbs as Medicine / 1

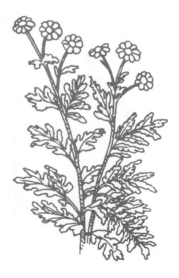

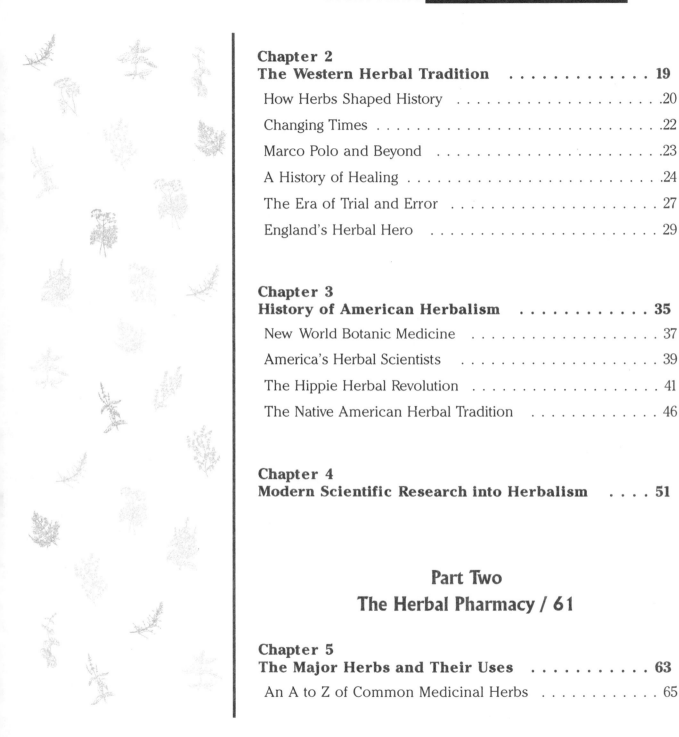

CONTENTS

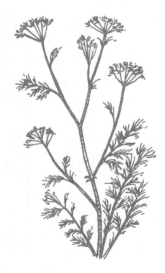

Part Three
Herbal Healing Today / 185

CONTENTS

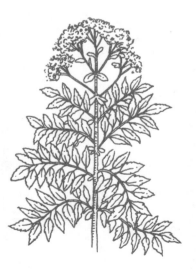

Acknowledgments

My profound thanks go to my dear friend Susan Shaw, who for the past 12 years has been general manager of the Morning Glory Natural Foods store in Nacogdoches, Texas, and who graciously consented to serve as my consultant on this book. Beginning as an avid organic gardener with an agricultural degree in soil science and management, Susan found her true calling in growing herbs and learning to use them for medicine before taking her talents public. Now, as the unofficial "herb wife" of an entire community, her store is a place where people interested in herbal remedies or other alternative methods of healing can find accurate information dispensed in a loving atmosphere. I could not have been more fortunate in having access to her vast knowledge and understanding of herbs and their uses while researching and writing this book. Thanks, Susie.

My research assistant, Kelly Calloway, a student at Stephen F. Austin University in Nacogdoches, has been an invaluable help. I am indebted to her not only for processing her way through dozens of Web sites to glean information and intuitively knowing just which books from the library would be helpful but also for being a hard and steady worker who never complained about what was sometimes a tedious chore. Quite truly, I could not have written this book without her help.

My heartfelt thanks go to my dear friend Jimmi Rushing, whose sophisticated knowledge of the world of the Internet and ability to access databases known only to the most elite researchers provided me with information I'd never have been able to obtain on my own—and who gave generously of her time and talent without thought of any more recompense than dispensing valuable information to those who need it.

My co author of *Love Planets* and fellow astrologer as well as close friend, Claudia Bader, provided me with a memorable phrase—and a good laugh when it was most needed.

Chris Santini, as always, was there for me when I needed to talk, to seek spiritual assistance, to reassure me that I'd get through the work even when I doubted myself.

And the feline inhabitants of my household—Princess Mushkin, Betsey Butterscotch, and Sylvester Albert, Lord Underfoot—were always on hand to remind me that life is about living, not about working.

Of course, it is necessary also to thank the spirits who both motivated the work and helped to process it through its many trials and tribulations. Writing a book is never easy—they made the task bearable when it seemed most difficult.

Introduction

The Herbal Renaissance

Herbs can perhaps point out a path for us on how we might grow and change in a big world that is becoming a global village. We know we can count on the safety and efficacy of herbs in ways that the latest drug can never achieve. We know that they reach out to us with their marvelous complexity and abilities to help us address the health problems of today, just as they addressed ancient ones. Herbs may be our best hope to bring the balance back between the healing forces and diseases.

—LINDA RECTOR PAGE, N.D., Ph.D., *Healthy Healing*

Herbs are booming. Earl Mindell, R. Ph., Ph.D., in his book *Herb Bible,* says that, "Perhaps the major reason for our renewed interest in herbalism can be attributed to the new emphasis on preventative medicine. The pendulum of science is on its return swing, and we now know that lifestyle and nutrition play significant roles in averting disease. There is a growing recognition that herbs, too, can play a vital role in promoting wellness. Unlike drugs, many herbs are taken as 'tonics,' that is, like many vitamins, they can be used primarily to maintain good health. Studies show that there are herbs that can reduce cholesterol, improve circulation, and even prevent cancer. Some herbs have been shown to enhance immune function, thus helping the body to fight against disease. Obviously, most of us would prefer to take an herb that would help us stay healthy than a drug when we are sick!"

The boom keeps on growing as the baby boomers begin to age and face the inevitable challenges of that process—menopause, prostate difficulties, weight gain, loss of memory, lack or energy, depression, and a host of other ails. From their youth, this generation was in revolt against the establishment, which included traditional, drug-based "Western" medicine. It wasn't long before some vegetarian hippies began growing

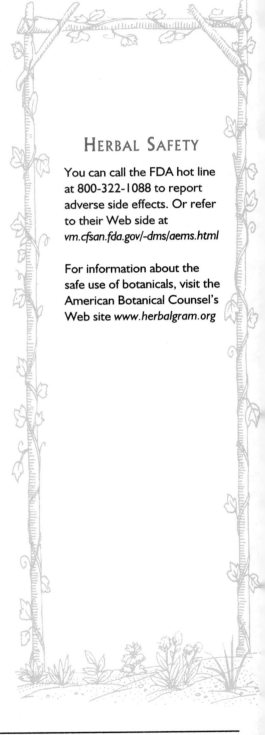

HERBAL SAFETY

You can call the FDA hot line at 800-322-1088 to report adverse side effects. Or refer to their Web side at *vm.cfsan.fda.gov/-dms/aems.html*

For information about the safe use of botanicals, visit the American Botanical Counsel's Web site *www.herbalgram.org*

their own food and in their quest for more natural living, eventually spawning the "back to the land" movement, adding herbs to their gardens and farm plots. The herbal renaissance was a movement that hitched a piggyback ride on a broader cultural shift.

It is the very lack of effective help from modern medicine that has led to the resurgence during the past decade of the popularity of herbal medicine, with its emphasis on nutrition and holistic treatment, especially as ailments caused by pollution and stress have continued to rise alarmingly—a development that has caused many people to turn to nature's herbs and other herbal products to help reverse the harmful effects of urban life.

Of course, humans have always used herbs medicinally: what was different was the *attitude* underlying the new surge of interest in herbs and herbal healing. A *paradigm shift* was taking place—a change in consciousness about the Earth and life on it. As the world shrunk in size, becoming a "global village," people began to see Earth as an intelligent being, evolving and growing just as did the humans who populated it.

In time it became apparent that the overprescribing of certain drugs—antibiotics in particular—had led to dire consequences: The pathogenic organisms that cause disease were mutating into drug-resistant strains at an alarming rate. Both the organisms and the diseases they cause were becoming more virulent while the human immune defense systems were becoming weakened by the use of pharmaceutical drugs—a billion-dollar industry that fed upon people's fear and desire for the "quick fix." "Doctor, I'm sick—give me a prescription for some pills," had been the ever-increasing demand.

The *symptoms* were often easy enough to relieve, but the danger was in the relief of symptoms without consideration of the underlying cause. Given instantaneous relief of what ailed them, people gradually gave up responsibility for their own health. The advantage of modern pharmacopoeia was that people could abdicate responsibility for how they lived their lives, for what they ate, and how much, for what they imbibed, and how much, for how they worked, and how much, for the games they played, and so forth. Unhealthy habits could be enjoyed, and their deleterious results could always be magically removed by a little colored pill. No need to develop *awareness* of one's own complexity—body, mind, emotions, and spirits, and how they interact. Someone else was trained to "know" what to do when you got into any kind of trouble. That the treatments didn't work—neither the medical nor the psychological—was easily ignored.

But when awareness grew that neither Dr. Daddy (nor Dr. Mom) could "fix" serious illnesses such as cancer, a cry went up for something else, something new—something *natural*.

Too many people were fed up with the "heroic" allopathic methods of treatment, from drugs to chemotherapy. The evidence that the latest scientific drugs weren't the answer was not only evident but glaring. The same scientific research that gave us the drugs was beginning to show that even the newest, most powerful antibiotics were effective for only about a year before the microbe or virus they were designed to kill or desist had mutated into a new strain against which the new drug was useless. The yearly flu shot, recommended especially for the young and the elderly and others who were vulnerable, was only effective against last year's flu.

Somebody, somewhere—actually a lot of people everywhere—said, "There's got to be a better way." And out of this dim dawning of consciousness there evolved a demand for treatment of disease and illness more in concert with the earth and its human inhabitants who were, at last, being seen as—not lords and masters of the universe—but common earthborn animals, just like sheep and dogs and cows and cats—and birds and fish and insects and bugs so small they cannot be seen. Yes, said this new realization, we humans are a part of Nature, not some strange God-created addition put here as its adversary.

Allopathic, or standard Western-type, medicine is called "heroic" because it was developed on the battlefields of the world over a long history of war; it is the calling of choice for the male population. And when one war or another was over, the doctors who had treated the wounded soldiers brought their heroic methods into the home and local hospital. Bleeding and purging were mere precursors to surgical removal of sick organs and the development of chemotherapy and other powerful, invasive "treatments" that as often killed as cured and often caused horrible side effects.

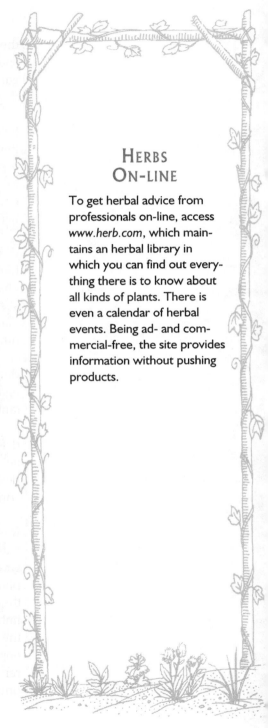

HERBS ON-LINE

To get herbal advice from professionals on-line, access *www.herb.com*, which maintains an herbal library in which you can find out everything there is to know about all kinds of plants. There is even a calendar of herbal events. Being ad- and commercial-free, the site provides information without pushing products.

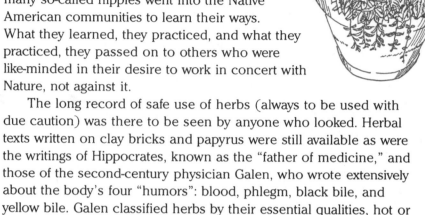

Fortunately, a few herbal healers had continued quietly and often in secret to carry on their old ways of herbal healing, keeping alive a long tradition and preserving a vast encyclopedia of knowledge. Many of these were indigenous peoples, and in the United States many so-called hippies went into the Native American communities to learn their ways. What they learned, they practiced, and what they practiced, they passed on to others who were like-minded in their desire to work in concert with Nature, not against it.

The long record of safe use of herbs (always to be used with due caution) was there to be seen by anyone who looked. Herbal texts written on clay bricks and papyrus were still available as were the writings of Hippocrates, known as the "father of medicine," and those of the second-century physician Galen, who wrote extensively about the body's four "humors": blood, phlegm, black bile, and yellow bile. Galen classified herbs by their essential qualities, hot or cold, dry or wet, and these theories were later expanded by seventh-century Arab physicians such as Avicenna, who was the most famous healer of his time.

Not satisfied with formal education alone, many of the '60s young began exploring on their own, learning more and more about herbs—how to grow them, how to prepare them, how to use them for healing. They began to see herbs as a spiritual path, not just a way to cure illnesses. This attitude was reflected in what they were learning from their Native American teachers and mentors.

As it became apparent that herbs were *dependable*—because, the reasoning went, they were *natural*—another movement arose, this one for *organic* plants to be used for food and medicine. After all, what use would herbs contaminated with pesticides be?

It wasn't long before entrepreneurial types all over began starting up companies to produce herbal products for the maintenance of health and the healing of ailments. A message had been sent and received: Appreciate the medicinal value of plants and preserve these finite resources in their native habitats. Field workers found countless herbs that had never been investigated for their healing properties, and they patiently worked with native peoples to glean their vast herbal knowledge and record it.

Healers began to pop up like jacks-in-the-box, using herbs and intuition in tandem. Psychology got into the act, too, as many of our physical ailments are intimately bound up with our emotional traumas. People began to understand themselves as whole beings, not a collection of parts. "I am not my liver, my spleen, my blood, nor my brain" was the paraphrase of the famous Buddhist doctrine. "I am all of me" was the new and often revolutionary statement being made by people of all ages.

Herbs are *universal*: They are the primary source of healing for the vast majority of the earth's population, and they do not discriminate between our bodies and our emotions. In fact, sometimes they work subtly on the emotional problem that is the root cause of the physical problem. In the most significant way, herbs are *holistic*—and very often herbalists insist that the whole plant be used for maximum effect. (Of course, there are plants whose effective parts are the leaves or roots, not both.)

As we enter the new millennium, the herbal renaissance is gathering force all around. It is breaking down the old divisions between traditional folk medicine and the modern scientific approach that depends so heavily on symptomatic relief. These two schools—so divergent in their attitudes toward health and healing—have much to learn from each other. We will all benefit if they eventually come together and act as one, despite their philosophical differences.

One sign of hope is that now modern science and technology have been put to use to study the herbal pharmacopoeia. Clearly, this is a sign of an enormous rebirth of interest in the ways of Nature and holistic healing. Researchers are finding that wild plants contain a storehouse of genetic information that may lead to new treatments for disease, especially those that have heretofore resisted treatment, such as AIDS and other immune deficiency diseases.

We are beginning to realize that to ignore Nature is to ask for trouble and that to ignore the nature of the *individual* courts failure in treating individuals, who, after all, are the ones receiving treatment. No matter how many studies are done in the laboratory on mice or other laboratory animals, and no matter how many

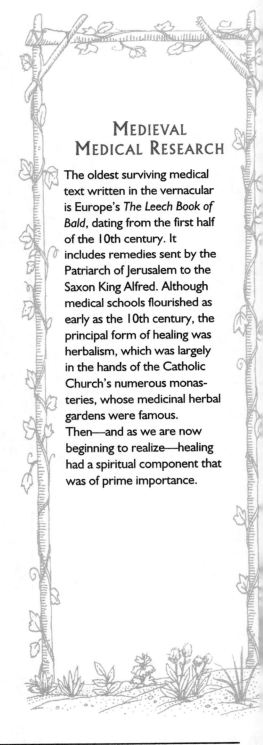

MEDIEVAL MEDICAL RESEARCH

The oldest surviving medical text written in the vernacular is Europe's *The Leech Book of Bald*, dating from the first half of the 10th century. It includes remedies sent by the Patriarch of Jerusalem to the Saxon King Alfred. Although medical schools flourished as early as the 10th century, the principal form of healing was herbalism, which was largely in the hands of the Catholic Church's numerous monasteries, whose medicinal herbal gardens were famous. Then—and as we are now beginning to realize—healing had a spiritual component that was of prime importance.

studies are done on groups of human beings, those results may not be applicable to you or to me. The lesson, however, of the vast complexity of the human species and of our natural environment has been appreciated by only a minority of researchers. These researchers realize that much more attention must be given to investigating the wealth of therapeutic possibilities that lie hidden in the secret vastness of Nature, who is not as unwilling to give up her secrets as we might fear. In reality, Nature's cures are there for the taking, if we pay attention and learn.

In recent years, innumerable books on herbs, herbal medicine, herbal remedies, and herbal preparations of all kinds, have rolled off the printing presses. The shelves of both libraries and bookstores are lined with them. Anyone with the desire to learn about these "miracle drugs" of nature has only to peruse the copious literature. In addition, there are numerous Web sites devoted to natural health.

This book is a simple yet comprehensive introduction to the wonders of herbal healing. Of course, it is impossible to even list the thousands of herbs that are known to exist, let alone "prescribe" for any single individual or specific ailment. It is up to each of us to do our own research, to learn to understand our own bodies and their peculiarities. The snag in the scientific method is that the intricacies of the individual human body are too varied and complex to be studied on an individual basis—and just as it is difficult to get a decision from a committee, it is difficult to prescribe for an individual based on studies done on people with no relationship to that particular individual.

True, the majority still hanker after the "magic bullet" that will cure them, and many scientists are still chasing this particular rainbow, looking for the new drug that will produce a pot of

gold. However, there are too many imponderables in the equation of what creates human health and how to maintain it, let alone how to treat what goes wrong with it, for science to ignore. As the great German philosopher Goethe wrote, "Nothing happens in living Nature that is not in relation to the whole." We do not have to be of a revolutionary persuasion philosophically to accept that the integration of man with Nature as a whole is a desirable end.

An old Chinese curse says, "May you be born in an interesting time," and these indeed are interesting times. But remember that the saying is a *curse*, which means we live also in difficult times. In a world that has long been dedicated to the pursuit of technological advancement and scientific exactness (even though that itself is an impossibility, as recent quantum physics has proved), a return to the most ancient form of medicine known to humankind is something of a shock. But there is no doubt that *herbal medicine is in the throes of a renaissance*. And it is probably fortunate that this much needed renaissance is coming at a time when there is the possibility of scientific validation of what has been intuitively and experientially known for centuries.

This book is divided into three parts. Part One covers the historical use of herbs as medicine from ancient beginnings to modern scientific research into herbal use as medicine. Part Two contains a selected listing of the major herbs in use today as well as an overview of herbal remedies from around the world, herbal therapies for common ailments, including in Chapter Five the components for your own "Herbal First Aid Kit," and a look at essential oils and herbal extracts and their uses. Part Three reviews herbal healing today and includes a guide to using herbs as medicinals safely, choices available, a guide to making your own herbal preparations, and a special section, "The Herbal Medicine Garden," for those who want to grow their own.

Part One

HISTORICAL USE OF HERBS AS MEDICINE

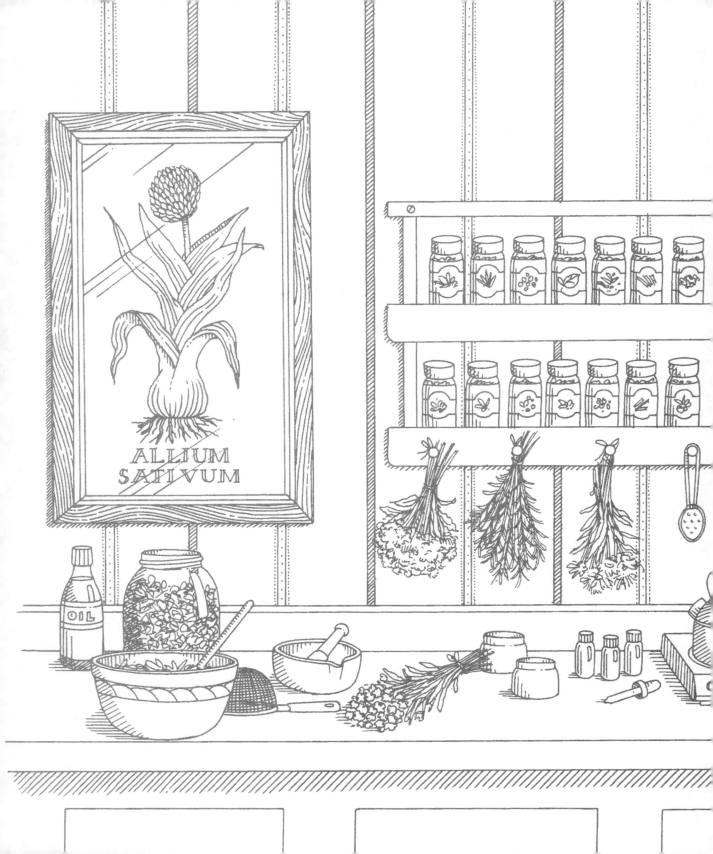

ALLIUM
SATIVUM

OIL

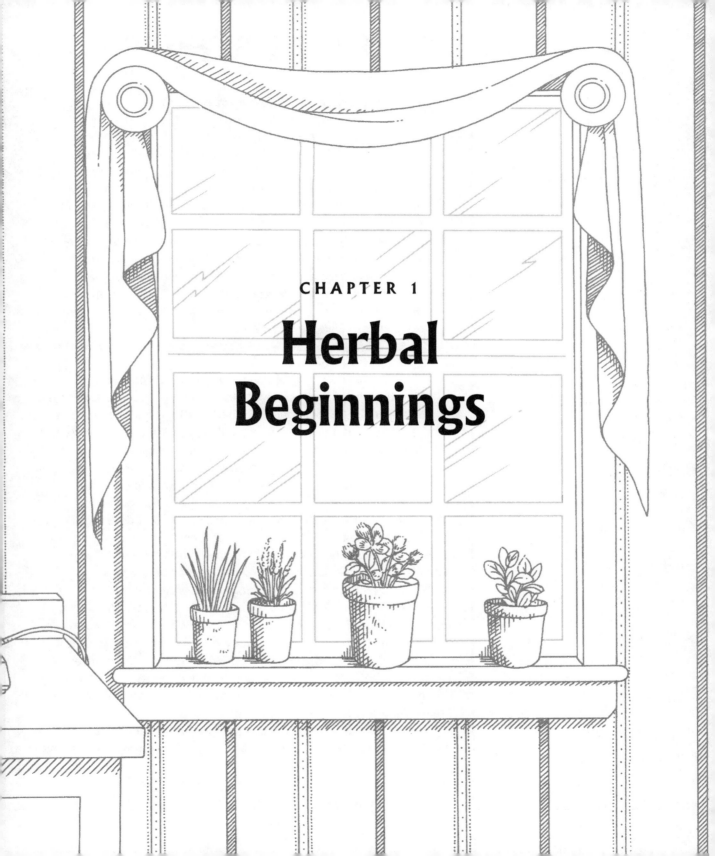

CHAPTER 1

Herbal Beginnings

Herbal medicine is the oldest form of therapy practiced by mankind, and much of this medicinal use of plants seems to have been based on a highly developed "dowsing" instinct, which led the healer of the tribe to the right plant and taught him or her its use. To a modern mind, the idea may seem bizarre, but wild animals certainly possess such an instinct, seeking out plants which will supply the nutrients they need and unerringly avoiding those which will poison them. These dowsing powers would explain the astonishing continuity of medicinal plant usage in the days before there were written records, or in tribes who have never known them, since the chain of oral tradition must have been broken over and over again by death, or by the scattering or obliteration of the tribe.

—BARBARA GRIGGS in *Green Medicine*

Humans have always depended on a close relationship with Nature. In order to survive, they needed to have an extensive knowledge of local plant life, both for food and medicine, and also for clothing and shelter. Humans also have usually lived closely with their work and farm animals, often even sharing living quarters with working animals such as oxen and horses. Naturally, since their own survival depended on the health of these work animals, they closely observed them. They watched sick sheep eat yarrow, lizards eat chamomile after being bitten by a snake, cats and dogs nibble grass and then vomit whatever had upset their stomachs, and many more such cases. The instincts of animals to derive benefits from plants is one of the most interesting facets of Nature at work.

We have learned more about native use of herbal remedies from explorers like Nicola Maxwell and modern-day ethnobotanists who have studied primitive herbal medicine than we have from anthropologists. This is because the shamanistic tradition—the world's oldest religion and its oldest medical profession—is still practiced in remote places, by tribes and peoples living in jungles, forests, and deserts. Though individual tribal practices vary widely, certain common threads run throughout.

Healing methods of indigenous peoples are generally gathered under the general term of *shamanism*, which is the religion of many traditional cultures throughout the world. Originating in central and northern Asia, it spread outward into the New World, Australia, Africa, and other parts of Asia. Shamanism speaks directly to the totality that encompasses all life and the environment, both terrestrial and celestial, in which that life resides and has its being. There is no separation of spirit and body, of human and animal/plant, of earth and cosmos.

Traditionally, tribal shamans have nurtured spiritual powers and brought them to a high degree of development, passing their knowledge and techniques along to succeeding generations. Wise in the lore of herbs and plants known to have healing properties, the shaman fused the practice of spiritual magic with the practice of healing. Indeed, there was no separation between the two—the practice of shamanism presupposes that we live in a psychospiritual as well as physical ecosystem. In this view, the entire world and all in it are imbued with spirit—all life is in communication at a deep level, beneath our awareness. Animals have their own type of consciousness and can know our thoughts and sense our feelings (as anyone with a pet cat or dog can attest).

Shamans believe they can transcend both time and space and, in so doing, avail themselves of the invisible powers that reside in the animal and vegetable kingdoms and in the elements—fire, earth, air, and water.

Nearly every such group has a shaman, or medicine man—or witch doctor—who is not only the chief medical advisor to the tribe but also its spiritual leader. His (or, sometimes, her) knowledge has been handed down to carefully chosen apprentices for generation after generation, and the secrets of the shamanistic practice are closely guarded. To enter into its elite ranks, a young aspirant must undergo great trials, both physically and psychologically, and must uphold strict ethical standards. The shamanistic tradition originated in Eurasia c. 4000 B.C.E. and spread across the world, to India, the Pacific, South America, and North America. The shaman was always a powerful personality with a pronounced gift for healing; in order to find the cure, he was supposedly able to travel in an out-of-body state to find the spirit

RECOMMENDED READING

For those interested in exploring the wide range of plants and their many uses employed by Native American Indians, here are some titles from the many books on the subject:

- *How Indians Use Wild Plants for Food, Medicine, and Crafts* by Frances Densmore
- *Cherokee Plants—Their Uses: A 400-Year-Old History* by Paul B. Hamel and Mary U. Chiltoskey
- *A Handbook of Northeastern Indian Medicinal Plants* by James A. Duke
- *Eastern/Central Medicinal Plants* by Stephen Foster and James A. Duke
- *The Herbal Medicine-Makers Handbook* by James Green
- *History, Myths, and Sacred Formulas of the Cherokees* by James Mooney

that was causing the illness. The tribe's shaman would also have had a highly developed instinct for herb dowsing and would have been the most important member of a community, trusted and revered by all. According to one African writer, the shaman was expected to be "trustworthy, upright morally, friendly, willing and ready to serve, able to discern people's needs, and not be exorbitant in their charges." Barbara Griggs comments that "this would have been a perfect description of the old-fashioned country doctor before the advent of the giant pharmaceutical companies and socialized medicine turned him into a harried and bureaucratized dispenser of pills."

The first "herbal guide" of which we have knowledge comes from Sumer, c. 5000 B.C.E. The Sumerians used herbs such as caraway and thyme for healing purposes. A surviving Egyptian text inscribed on papyri dating to c. 1700 B.C.E. records that many common herbs, such as garlic and juniper, were used medicinally for the previous 4000 years, and herbal prescriptions have been found written in hieroglyphics on other papyri from ancient Egypt.

By the time of Hippocrates (468–377 B.C.E.), the herbal tradition had absorbed ideas from Eastern traditions, such as from Assyria and India, making Indian herbs—such as ginger and basil—highly prized. Hippocrates categorized all foods and herbs by fundamental qualities, relating these to the elements—fire, earth, air, and water—which were essential components to the study of astrology (which at the time was part of medicine).

Thus, the early Greeks saw the world as composed of the four elements, and the elements were related to the seasons. Each element was related to one of the four fundamental qualities—bodily fluids or "humors"—and to four types of temperaments. It was thought that one of the humors was dominant in each individual and would therefore affect the personality and the health problems likely to be encountered.

Today, astrology bears out these ancient tenets—as it did then. In the following section, you will find a specially designed method that will enable you to discover your own type, the knowledge of which will help you to choose herbal remedies most appropriate for your individual personality and your particular tendencies toward certain ailments.

Your Healing Type

Your healing type is imprinted at the moment of birth by the elemental distribution of your inborn nature. Harmonizing with your personal element makeup is an excellent way both to prevent illness and to augment or restore health. The elements represent our "personal weather," both emotionally and physically.

There are four basic types, again, related to fire, earth, water, and air. You may be a single type, a mixture of two types, or a multiple type. Also, you may find emphasis on one type or another (especially if you are a mixed type) at different times of the month, day, year, or over a lifespan.

First you must find out your natural affinity for each of the four elements; you will use this information to determine your type. Then you can tune in to your basic type and learn to work with its healing energy.

Treat this exercise like a game and have fun with it.

Discovering Your Healing Type

From the word lists that follow rate the degree—ALWAYS, OFTEN, RARELY, or NEVER—to which the word applies to you. The idea is for you to make contact with your deep inner self's order or innate elemental pattern. Choose a different colored pencil for each of the four words, for example, the color red for ALWAYS, blue for OFTEN, and so on. You may find that you are consistently choosing the same color or colors for words from a particular list or for certain words or groups of words. Try not to think or decide what color goes with which words; just let the process flow from your interior self until you have finished. You don't have to work in any particular order; go back and forth between the lists if you like.

One suggestion is to first read a list quickly and spontaneously choose words that produce a strong emotional charge, either positive—ALWAYS—or negative—NEVER—and afterward go back and rate those that fall into the OFTEN or RARELY categories.

HEALING AND SELF-HEALING

Ancient peoples understood that all healing was ultimately self-healing, something now being widely recognized, as this quotation from the well-known psychologist Lawrence LeShan, writing in *The Utne Reader*, aptly demonstrates.

Healing ultimately occurs with self-healing. The best surgeon in the world knows that all you can do is bring the ends of a surgical wound together cleanly and precisely and let nature heal the patient. The whole problem of healing is arranging for this to happen. Sometimes you have to remove something like a splinter, a virus, or bacteria that is damaging the patient, something the patient's self-healing abilities can't handle themselves. Then you try to arrange a climate in which the patient's self-healing abilities work to the fullest.

Fire, Earth, Water, Air Types

FIRE	EARTH	WATER	AIR
Self-starting	Organized	Feeling	Communicative
Self-confident	Serious	Sensitive	Quick-witted
Action-initiating	Practical	Sympathetic	Inquisitive
Decisive	Down-to-earth	Nostalgic	Adaptable
Outgoing	Realistic	Comfort-loving	Curious
Forceful	Ambitious	Security-oriented	Versatile
Driving	Hardworking	Domestic	Flexible
Active	Structured	Family-oriented	Variety-seeking
Strong	Disciplined	Food-oriented	Relationship-oriented
Adventurous	Analytical	Emotional	Cooperative
Self-expressive	Detail-oriented	Intense	Sociable
Self-aware	Methodical	Passionate	Companionable
Dramatic	Sensible	Secretive	Just
Playful	Sanitary	Mysterious	Balanced
Fun-loving	Stable	Compassionate	Tolerant
Powerful	Steady	Benevolent	Impartial
Impressive	Reliable	Sentimental	Intellectually detached
Enthusiastic	Productive	Intuitive	Friendly
Expansive	Persistent	Escapist	Innovative
Optimistic	Determined	Spacey	Independent
Generous	Deliberate	Impractical	Original
Outgoing	Money-oriented	Unrealistic	Individualistic
Blunt	Prudent	Artistic	Nonconformist
Outdoors-oriented	Cautious	Inspired	Charming
Travel-oriented	Economical	Receptive	Refined
Careless	Self-controlled	Moody	Studious
Explosive	Reserved	Clinging	Babbling
Foolhardy	Pessimistic	Brooding	Nervous
Egotistical		Emotionally perceptive	Superficial
		Passive	Mentally organized

If you choose words *only* from a single list, you are a pure type (this is rare). Most people will have at least a few words from at least two elemental categories. To determine your type, first count the words *from each list* that you have placed into each column. The highest number of words from any one list in your ALWAYS column determines your *primary type*.

For example, if you choose 20 words from the Fire category and placed them in the ALWAYS column but placed a lower number from any or all the other lists in ALWAYS, you are a basic fire type. Having determined your primary type, next count the words in your OFTEN column. If the highest number of these words comes from the *same* element as those in your ALWAYS column, more emphasis is placed upon the primary type.

If, however, an equal or greater number of words comes from a *different* list, you have a secondary type. For example, if you are a basic fire type but have your highest number in the OFTEN category from the water list, you are a mixed fire-water type.

The third step is to determine if you have a missing or inferior (de-emphasized) element. To do this, follow the same procedure outlined above for the NEVER category, which will indicate the missing element if there is one; then follow the procedure for the RARELY category, which will indicate the inferior element.

A missing or de-emphasized (RARELY) element means that there is an imbalance; ideally, all four elements would be represented. When an imbalance occurs (and it is common), the missing element can be "added" by consciously seeking to tune in to it. For example, if Earth is missing, then "earth-grounding" can be added by planting a garden, working with the hands, or just sitting on the ground and tuning into Mother Nature. Similarly, water can be added by going to the seaside or lakeshore, taking long soaks in the tub, or walking in the rain.

Sometimes, we get elementally out of balance—such might be the case when a water type is forced to go on a camping trip in the mountains or, conversely, an air type has to spend time in the wet air of a lakeside or beside the ocean. When imbalance occurs, and the stress of ordinary living can cause this to happen, illness can follow. The best way to counteract this is to rebalance ourselves elementally. Your elemental balance provides important clues to the maintenance of health and the means of healing. Allowing ourselves to be "in our element" is a wonderful curative.

THE ORIGINAL "WONDER DRUG"

An Egyptian papyrus written c. 1500 B.C.E., called the *Papyrus Ebers*, (after Georg Ebers the Egyptologist who discovered it) refers to more than 700 plants that served as medicines. The plants include peppermint, myrrh, and castor oil. One of the earliest known medical textbooks, the *Papyrus Ebers* tells the physician to apply a piece of moldy bread to an open wound. As we know today, the "wonder drug" we call penicillin was discovered accidentally by Sir Alexander Fleming in 1928—thousands of years after the Egyptians knew of its antibiotic qualities! Sir Fleming, working in his laboratory, just happened to notice that bread mold was a potent antibiotic. That chance observation led to the development of penicillin and a whole range of "new" drugs that were actually as old as the pyramids!

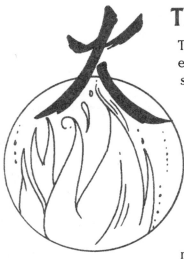

The Fire Type

The energy of fire is radiant. Your energy is flowing and you are excitable, enthusiastic, impatient, spontaneous, quick to react, self-centered, overly objective. Your natural high spirits give you self-esteem. Strength comes in spurts. A strong desire for self-expression and the need for freedom are your dominant characteristics.

Being cooped up depletes your life force; you need vigorous physical activity during the daytime, preferably out in the sunshine, with as much contact with the sun as possible. Winter in cold climates is hard on you, but sufficient outdoor activity during the hot summer months will allow you to store your elemental energy against the gloom of indoor winter months. Your energy goes down when the sun does. Early to bed, early to rise is a good health habit.

Illness, which can be brought on by over-excitement and a lack of proper rest, is a problem for you as you dislike being confined and inactive. You need to develop patience with illness or infirmity; premature return to activity can bring on a relapse. Restore balance by incorporating sunlight into your healing process. You are prone to the syndrome known as SAD, or seasonal affective disorder, caused by lack of sunlight. Light treatment can help.

You tend to suffer from headaches, injuries resulting from impulsive behavior, heart problems due to overwork and overactivity, and chronic back pain, often the product of lack of rest.

When ill or recovering, other fire types are healing for you as they replenish your energy. Air types are good but can tire you with their endless mental speculations. Avoid earth and water types; earth smothers you; water drenches your fire.

Some herbal remedies that will help to renew you include heather, for self-centeredness; impatiens, for lack of patience; hornbeam, for mental and physical exhaustion; and vervain, for tension and stress.

The Earth Type

The energy of earth is related closely to the physical plane and senses. Your energy is stable and you are patient, reliable, hard-working, commonsensical, practical, and stubborn, and have extra-ordinary stamina. The desire for concrete results and the self-discipline needed to get them are your dominant characteristics.

You need to be in physical contact with your element, to get your hands and feet into the soil, handle growing things and the solid basic material of the earth, such as rocks and minerals. Crystal therapy often works wonders for earth types.

Though you have great physical stamina, you are not inclined to physical exertion and need to push yourself to exercise regularly. You need to go at your own pace, especially in the matter of sleeping and waking. Being rushed can make you ill, literally, or delay recovery. When ill, you recuperate slowly but steadily and thoroughly. Pragmatic even when ill, you are a serene patient *if* you are convinced the treatment will produce concrete results.

You tend to have throat problems, get colds with sore throats as a result of emotional congestion or pushing your endurance level beyond its limit by continuing to work long past time to rest. You are prone to digestive upsets resulting from nerves and your desire for perfection. Bones can be brittle—women especially need to guard against osteoporosis—and teeth can cause problems. Regular dental checkups are a must. Skin, too, is sensitive and can become dry and scaly if not cared for properly. Restore balance by cultivating your sensuous side not only when ill but also as a preventive measure. Massage and scented body lotions are good choices.

When ill or recovering, fire people energize you, and water types soothe you. Other earth types can make the atmosphere too heavy. Avoid air types whose lack of common sense annoys you.

Some herbal remedies that will help to renew you include beech, to combat self-criticism; chicory, for possessiveness; mustard, for melancholy; and oak, for heavy responsibilities.

HERBS IN BIBLICAL TIMES

In Genesis, we are told that "on the third day of creation God said, 'Let the earth bring forth grass, the herb yielding seed, and the fruit tree yielding fruit after his kind, whose seed is in itself upon the earth: and it was so.'"

Both the Old and the New Testaments contain numerous references to commonly used herbs from biblical times.

Herbs such as cinnamon, pomegranate bark, aloe, garlic, onions, cloves, and saffron are mentioned in the Bible, and numerous references make it apparent that the ancient Hebrews had an enduring reverence for plants as medicine. In Ecclesiastes, we are advised that "the Lord created medicines from the earth, and a sensible man doesn't despise them."

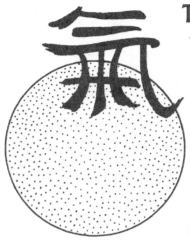

The Air Type

The energy of air is ephemeral. Your energy is constantly shifting and you are abstract, detached, fair-minded, talkative, diplomatic, and multifaceted. A preference for detachment from the "messy" human emotions and the emphasizing of theory and concepts are your dominant characteristics.

Prolonged contact with wet air depletes you, and in a humid climate, you should have a dehumidifier in your room. You find emotional display upsetting; an atmosphere heavy with emotion can make you ill. Witnessing or coping with outbursts of weeping or temperament can bring on exhaustion. You prefer to talk about emotions rationally rather than actually dealing with them, but repressing your own emotions can cause illness.

You have nervous energy and need to dissipate it with mental activity in order to get a good night's sleep. Allow sufficient winding down time before bed; it's a good time to spend a quiet half-hour in meditation. It's important for you to maintain a calm restful environment to counteract your inclination to live in your busy head.

When ill, you want to know everything about what ails you and research your diagnosis extensively, talking to everyone involved in your health care. Though you hate being confined to bed, you can deal with it if you have plenty of mental stimulation in a calm, unemotional atmosphere. Restore balance by frequent breathing exercises.

You are susceptible to respiratory ailments, especially those affecting the lungs, such as pneumonia. You are likely to throw out a shoulder, injure your hands (carpal tunnel syndrome is a risk) and arms, suffer a broken hip, or sprain an ankle. Kidney problems and circulation difficulties can arise.

When ill or recovering, fellow air types provide the mental stimulation and empathy you need. Fire types are energizing. Avoid earth types, as you find their practicality depressing, and water types, whose emotionality gets on your nerves.

Some herbal remedies that will help to renew you include agrimony, for worry underneath the cheerfulness; olive, for mental fatigue; white chestnut, for persistent mental arguments and conversations; and wild oat, for indecision and endlessly reviewing options.

THE FOUR HUMORS

In the original Greek system, each type was associated with a different temperament, fluid, season, and temperature as follows:

FIRE
Temperament = Choleric
Fluid = Yellow bile
Season = Summer
Temperature = Dry

The choleric temperament was considered to be hot and dry, a natural conclusion for fire. It was associated with a hot temper and liver disorders (the liver is supposed to be the seat of the emotions). Cool and moist plants were used to balance fire types.

WATER
Temperament = Phlegmatic
Fluid = Phlegm
Season = Winter
Temperature = Cold and Damp

The nature of the phlegmatic person was considered to be cold. Typical illnesses were those involving phlegm, or respiratory and chest problems. Warm and dry herbs were preferred to restore balance.

AIR
Temperament = Sanguine
Fluid = Blood
Season = Spring
Temperature = Damp

The person with a sanguine temperament was considered ideal—the word means equable or even—but also was inclined to self-indulgence, which meant that gout and an upset digestive system were the usual problems. Cool, dry herbs were recommended for balance.

EARTH
Temperament = Melancholic
Fluid = Black bile
Season = Fall
Temperature = Cold and Dry

The person with a melancholic nature was considered to be cold and dry. Typical illnesses included depression or gloominess, and constipation. Treatment was with hot herbs, which would affect balance.

Aromatic herbs have been used since antiquity for cleansing and healing both mind and body. Records from the East tell us that distilleries were employed as long ago as c. 5000 B.C.E. for the extracting of aromatic waters and essential oils. These were used extensively during ceremonies, including the healing ceremony. No distinction was made between spiritual and physical illness. Even today, some religious ceremonies, like the Catholic Mass, use incense in their ritual, a practice that harks back to the most ancient of human activities.

The Water Type

The energy of water is flowing. You are sensitive, intuitive, emotional, psychic, imaginative, and insecure, and various intangibles play a large part in your life. Being exquisitely tuned in to feelings—your own and other people's—and being very aware of your unconscious processes, which you access through dreams and intuition, are your dominant characteristics.

Although your feeling responses can go from extreme compassion to total self-pity, you trust your inner promptings and act on them. When your feelings are blocked or repressed, you can suffer psychosomatic ailments. You need to express feelings freely; if they stay inside, they solidify into resentment and a bad temper, which can bring on ill health. When upset, you can restore balance by lying in a warm bath until feelings have settled.

Your inner landscape is forever in flux, like the ocean tides. Waves of feeling wash over you constantly; if they are not expressed, trouble results. Do not accept criticism for being irrational, emotional, or overly sensitive.

Insisting on the right to express feelings in a nonjudgmental atmosphere will allow you to maintain your inner harmony and physical health. You need time and space to yourself. Privacy and frequent isolation can help you to sort out your complicated feelings so that you can deal with stress.

When ill, you need a quiet, calm atmosphere and plenty of sleep to promote dreaming. You respond to a spiritual environment. Meditation and prayer come easily and are of utmost importance in your healing process, which can be accelerated by soft music, preferably strings, and being near water—an ocean or a lake. Hot springs are also good. Many of your complaints are vague in nature and respond to a total-body immersion.

THE HOLISTIC TRADITION

Indigenous peoples all over the world for whom shamanism was a way of life were not merely brilliant herbalists. They were not "rational" in the sense of today's scientist, who strives for total objectivity, but were "holistic." Native peoples understood instinctively— and experientially—that mind, body, and spirit were inseparable, that illness in one produced illness in the others. Their view of nature was pantheistic—an attitude that holds that every animal, plant, tree, and all other aspects of nature were invested with spiritual life.

You can suffer immune system disorders, breast lumps, fluid retention, constipation, reproductive-system complaints, foot problems, and glandular imbalance.

When ill or recovering, you benefit from the practical nature of earth types. Other water types are sympathetic but feed your self-pity. Avoid fire, which boils the water nature, and air, which lacks empathy.

Some herbal remedies that will help to renew you include clematis, for excess dreaminess; honeysuckle, for overcoming nostalgic obsession; mimulus, for fear and anxiety; and walnut, for oversensitivity to the influence of others.

The Mixed Types

If you are a mixed type, read the descriptions that follow. You can compare how each of the two elements relates to each or the other *within you* by referring to the previous discussions of the pure types and how they relate to each other.

Fire/Earth

You mix practicality with impracticality, impulsiveness with patience. You can be the most reliable of persons, yet suddenly go off without notice. You can make the visionary real. You mix strength and courage. Trouble results when you are insensitive to your environment, become self-centered to the point of hypochondria, or fail to take proper health measures or precautions.

Fire/Air

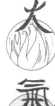

You put ideas into action, join vision to logic. You are objective but can be affectionate as well. You like to gain knowledge about your own health and will seek out appropriate treatment from an intellectual standpoint. Trouble results when you disconnect from your spiritual needs and concentrate too narrowly on the intellectual level or when you exhaust yourself through restlessness and unrealistic adventures.

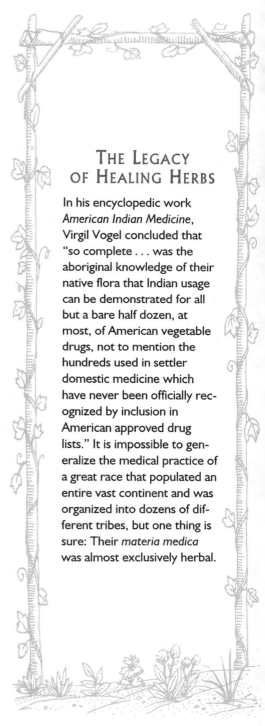

THE LEGACY OF HEALING HERBS

In his encyclopedic work *American Indian Medicine*, Virgil Vogel concluded that "so complete . . . was the aboriginal knowledge of their native flora that Indian usage can be demonstrated for all but a bare half dozen, at most, of American vegetable drugs, not to mention the hundreds used in settler domestic medicine which have never been officially recognized by inclusion in American approved drug lists." It is impossible to generalize the medical practice of a great race that populated an entire vast continent and was organized into dozens of different tribes, but one thing is sure: Their *materia medica* was almost exclusively herbal.

Fire/Water

You are the most intuitive of the mixed types. You're very fluid, and your connection to your inner realm is amazing. You get accurate hunches about what's wrong with you if you feel ill. Impressionable and sensitive, you respond well to visualizations to promote health and healing. Trouble results when you succumb to hysteria and over-emotionalism or wall yourself off in your own private universe.

Earth/Air

You are extremely efficient, combining objectivity with practicality, and you are likely to be involved in your own health and health care, using conventional means of treatment for illness while being open to unorthodox methods. You plan and execute well and are in a position to stay on top of a situation. Trouble results when you fall prey to skepticism, pessimism, or a cynical view of life.

Earth/Water

You are simultaneously sensitive and grounded, both intuitive and practical. You have a talent for accepting whatever cards life deals you and making them work. When ill, you tend to feel your way into your own depths to find the cure. Trouble results when you overindulge, which can produce addictions, or use your depths as a means of escape from harsh reality.

Air/Water

You are extremely sensitive, combining compassionate feeling with objectivity. You can detach from your emotions and empathetic responses and analyze your experience coolly. With both a logical mind and the ability to feel, you can affect the course of any illness from both angles. Trouble results when you rely too heavily on your intellectual abilities, which makes you high-strung and nervous.

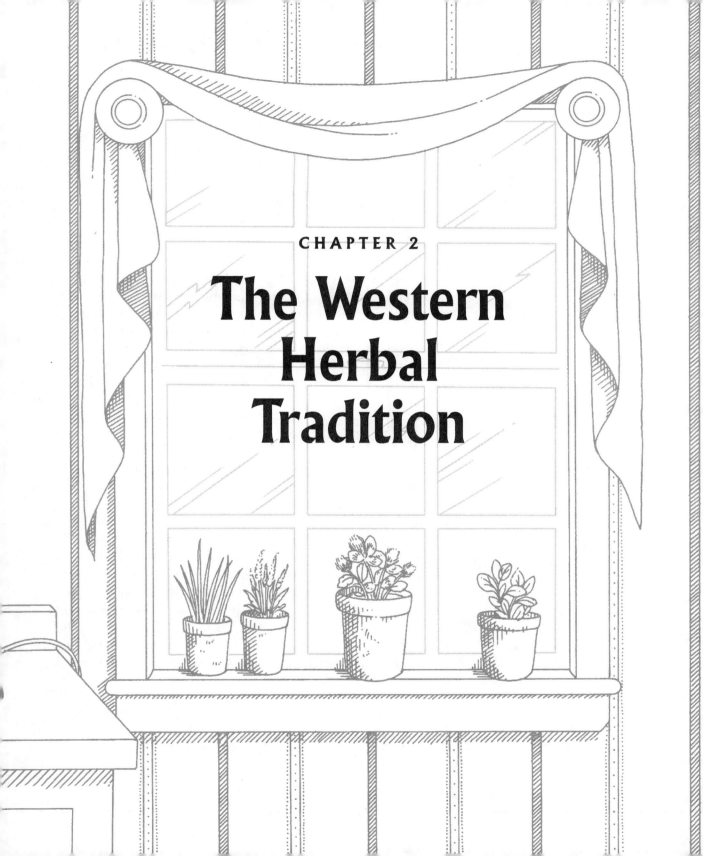

CHAPTER 2

The Western Herbal Tradition

The Lord hath created medicines out of the earth;
and he that is wise will not abhor them.
                    —Apocrypha, Ecclesiasticus 34:4

Why should a man die, who has sage in his garden?
        —Anon, Regimen Sanitatis Salernitanum, Medieval Herbal

Eighteen centuries before the advent of Christianity, Joseph was sold by his brothers to "a company of Ishmaelites coming from Gilead, with their camels bearing spicery and balm and myrrh, going to carry it down to Egypt." The history of Western herbal medicine begins with the history of the spice trade. Like rivers of fragrance that converted themselves into rivers of money, all the spices of the East—pepper, poppy seed, ginger, cloves, sesame, nutmeg, mace, turmeric, cinnamon, and basil—to name only a portion of this vast commerce, poured down the Nile River and across the hot desert sands.

How Herbs Shaped History

For many thousands of years, these seemingly insignificant curls of bark, shriveled seeds, dried leaves, and gnarled roots flowed along the trade route of antiquity—be they watery or sandy—into human history, which shaped their uses from sacred and ceremonial to magical and medicinal, from ritualistic incenses and fragrant perfumery to the simple, aromatic uses of the hearth and home remedies for a variety of human ailments, ills, and adverse conditions.

More than 3000 years ago, the Arab traders—monopolists of the coveted flow of herbs and spices from East to West—kept their sources of supply deeply secret, telling dark and scary stories to their potential rivals of the dangers that lurked in the distant lands of India, China, Java, and points beyond, from whence their precious products originated.

Their laden caravans—some with as many as four thousand camels—were loaded with the rich treasures of the East, including spices more valuable than gold. These products made their way from Goa, Calicut, and the Orient to the eager markets of

Nineveh and Babylon, and thence to Carthage, Alexandria, and Rome. And wherever herbs and spices were traded, their purveyors were enriched beyond the fantastic imaginings of the *Arabian Nights*.

The ships of the Phoenicians carried a vast array of merchandise, departing from Tyre, their richest and busiest port. The Bible tells us that they traded "of all spices," and it is thought that the famed King Solomon, c. 1000 B.C.E., made his great wealth mainly from spices and herbs. By agreement with the Phoenician king, Hiram, King Solomon built the ships in which the Phoenicians and Israelites sailed in search of these costly plant products. And when the beauteous and powerful Queen of Sheba visited Solomon, she brought him as a gift, "a very great train, with camels that bear spices." The queen had them in plenty to give, for Sheba is the ancient name for today's Yemen, believed by the Greeks and Romans to be the home of spices.

However, because of the intense secretiveness of the Arab traders, the buyers of Greece and Rome knew as little about the actual origins of their products as they did about the as yet to be discovered New World. They had a notion that somewhere there were lands beyond even fabled India, which produced spices and herbs as well as other commodities such as gold and tin. Pliny the Elder the Roman historian and naturalist, tells us that the first Roman emperor, Augustus, sent an expedition to Arabia in an attempt to discover the sources and routes of the wily Arab merchants, who, coerced by the force of the Romans, gave directions that led them through the vast desolate and waterless desert, and they were lucky to return alive. Needless to say, they did not discover the secret trade routes of the Arabs.

Having discovered that the overland route was treacherous and deadly, Roman ships took to following the Arabian and Indian shoreline—which, although it had greater speed to recommend it, was equally fraught with danger from storm, shipwreck, and pirate raids. Finally, in the days of Tiberius Caesar, at the beginning of the Christian era, Rome's sailors discovered how to use the monsoons, those seasonal winds that blow east in summer and west in winter off of the Indian Ocean. Pushed by these friendly forces, their ships—loaded with the precious spices and herbs—could reach the great markets of Europe with amazing speed.

ANCIENT HEALING HERBS

The plants we know as healing herbs were on Earth before humans evolved. No one knows how long it took for humanity to discover the curative power of plants or how it came about, but prehistoric sites in Iraq show that the Neanderthals used yarrow, marsh mallow, and other healing herbs some 60,000 years ago. Possibly prehistoric people noticed that when ill, animals ate particular plants they did not otherwise consume. Being curious, no doubt, people began to experiment with these plants, thus discovering that they produced certain effects. For example, perhaps they caused sleepiness or wakefulness or increased urine output, helped constipation, or stopped diarrhea, eased pain, or lifted the spirits. The effective herbs were then incorporated into the shamanistic practices of the time (shamans were the first medical practitioners on Earth).

These markets were great indeed; during the early centuries of Christianity, under Roman rule, European cities enjoyed great wealth. Spices were of such high value because of their many merits; they could be used to preserve food, heal wounds, and treat illnesses, and were an essential part of sacred ceremonial events, such as the crowning and burial of emperors. Tacitus reports that Nero's wife Poppaea, who died in A.D. 65, was buried with an entire year of Rome's cinnamon supply.

Then, the barbarians, who had been knocking loudly at Rome's gates during the days of banquets, debaucheries, and circuses in the great Colosseum, broke through. With their arrival, the glory days— the virtues as well as the vices—of European civilization ended. Religion, art, law, and science stood still, and navigation and commerce among nations virtually vanished.

Changing Times

By the end of the 7th century, papyrus from Egypt had disappeared from Europe's markets and, along with it, the spices and the wealth they generated. As darkness settled over Western Europe, a new religion was spawned at Mecca by a camel driver named Mohammed, who married the widow of a wealthy Arabian spice trader. The new religion of Islam was spread throughout Asia. The missionaries gathered spices and herbs and spread knowledge of their use everywhere they went. When, in 711, the Mohammedan Moors conquered Spain they brought with them not only the East's vast learning but also its taste for luxury, including its appetite for spices. In the wake of the invasion of Spain, the winds of trade once more blew against Europe's shores.

By the 10th century, Venice, which had been founded 500 years earlier as a refuge from the barbarians invading from the north, developed a great merchant fleet, which she defended with warships. The Venetian merchants sailed their galleys laden with sacks of spices worth 200,000 ducats and kept a stranglehold on the commerce in Western waters. And they grew fabulously rich in the process.

In the Middle Ages in Europe, a pound of ginger bought a sheep, and a pound of mace bought three sheep or half a cow. Pepper was almost priceless; it was counted out berry by berry just as prescription pills are carefully counted today. Pepper was so valuable that in medieval France, a pound of it could buy a serf his freedom.

Despite the new trade, Europeans by and large did not know the sources from which the precious plant products derived. During the Crusades, feudal lords and rich merchants went to war not only to carry the cross and wrest the Holy Land from the "infidel" Moslems, but also to locate the sources of the precious spices for which they had an ever-increasing desire. But the Crusaders returned with as little knowledge of the spice lands as had their Roman antecedents centuries earlier.

Marco Polo and Beyond

Nine crusades intermingled East with West, and overland routes through the Alps to Germany and France were developed as well as waterways through Gibraltar to Brugge, Southampton, and London ports. However, a more momentous journey, in 1271, was that of the Polo brothers Nicolo and Maffeo, who headed not for Palestine but for "Cathay," or China. Upon their return, Nicolo took his 17-year-old son Marco with him on the next journey—which lasted for 24 years. Marco Polo was 41 when he came home to Venice and told his fascinating tales of what he had seen on his travels. These tales became the first link in a chain of great events: the downfall of Venice's monopoly on Western merchant trade, the end of the Arab monopoly on the spice trade, the discovery of the New World, and the opening of direct trade with the Orient.

Although a new period of darkness ensued with the fall of the Tartar dynasty when China turned its back on the West and closed itself off from trade with Europe, making Cathay impregnable, a young Genoese sea captain read in Latin *The Book of Marco Polo* and pondered how one might now reach the marvels of which the intrepid adventurer had written. It was the middle of the 14th century when Christopher Columbus daringly decided to sail not east but west, thereby discovering the New World, in search of pepper and other spices and herbs.

BENEDICTINE BLESSINGS

The Benedictine monks were among the most skilled of medieval herbalists. Their herb gardens so impressed the emperor Charlemagne that he declared a law requiring all the monasteries in his realm to plant "physic gardens." The most famous Benedictine herbalist was St. Hildegard of Bingen (1078–1179) who wrote *Hildegard's Medicine*, a compilation of early German folk medicine with her own expert knowledge gained from growing and using herbs. At a time of general illiteracy, Hildegard was unique. She was a learned woman who was both monk and writer. If she had not recorded the herbal information she possessed, much of that knowledge would have died with her.

Pepper became a metaphor for the wealth that could be had from seafaring, and one April morning in 1788, the 100-ton brig *Cadet* sailed out of Salem's harbor, the first of over a thousand "pepper voyages" undertaken by Americans over the next 85 years.

Meanwhile, the colonists, short of medical supplies and waiting for the ships to come home, began to explore the indigenous plants they found on these shores, often with guidance from Native Americans, who were already learned in the medicinal uses of their native plants.

A History of Healing

The healing properties of plants have not changed in these thousands of years (healing herbs of the ancient world are still healing herbs today). Called "green medicine," herbs were treated with respect for their healing and curative powers. Those who practiced herbal healing spent much of their time in the fields gathering their "simples," as herbs were called. They learned when the best times were to harvest different herbs—whether in the morning, late afternoon, or at eventide, or during specific phases of the moon. From earliest times, the influence of the moon on plants was considered extremely important. The moon represented a deep and visible source of connectedness with the world of Nature, and an extension of Nature's products, both plant and animal. It is no wonder that early herbalists were almost always women—traditionally women were the fundamental guardians of elemental energy. They maintained the hearth fires, presided over the drawing of well water, and saw to the maintenance of the dwelling place. The moon's visible cycle in the sky matched women's own inner, invisible 28-day cycle, so women were thought to be connected to and represented by the moon and her phases, which were of prime importance to agricultural cultures.

These early herbalists kept careful records of the herbs they gathered, dried, combined, and prescribed. Explicit instructions were given as to the time of day and year during which any given herbal remedy would be most effective. Herbs have always been related to the practice of magic, which was actually nothing more than wise women's knowledge of the natural world and of the plants they

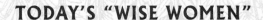

TODAY'S "WISE WOMEN"

Michael Castleman, author of *The Healing Herbs*, states flatly that "even in the United States most people view physicians as the health-care choice of last resort." He says that although the medical profession promotes the idea that family doctors are our primary providers, "studies show that before people call health professionals, *about 90 percent* consult a friend or family member, and those 'health advisers' are overwhelmingly women."

Not only have women been the primary *providers* of health care for most of the world for eons, they are the primary *consumers* of health care, now as then. Women have always had the responsibility for the health of their families—husbands and children as well as the elderly in an extended family. Even today, nearly half of all visits to physicians are made by women, who receive $^3/_4$ of all prescriptions.

Given these historical facts, it is no surprise that there is a large number of herbs that have traditionally been used to treat womanly concerns—to calm the womb, to induce conception, to trigger menstruation, to ease the pain of childbirth, to promote health in a pregnant woman, to induce abortion, to increase lactation or dry it up. In addition, women's concerns were for childhood ailments, such as infant colic and infectious diarrhea, a leading cause of infant death still today in undeveloped countries. Because these were the daily concerns of women patients, they became the focus of women healers' work.

These women healers were themselves wives and mothers, aunts and grandmothers—members of families. In those days, ordinary people had the knowledge to treat themselves. They used their own supplies, from their larders and their gardens, or foraged for wild plants growing in nearby fields and meadows, or in the hills. There may have been a local "doctor," who was called on in times of dire emergency, but for the most part, for common ailments, treatment was home-based. And, of course, the women healers were part of the home and hearth.

gathered and studied. These herbal healers passed on their knowledge from generation to generation, first orally and then in written "prescription" manuals or in daily journals of their activities and investigations into the properties of different plants and herbs.

Herbs also have a long connection to astrology, and until fairly recent times, medicine and astrology were studied together. Nostradamus, like many of history's wise men, was an astrologer as well as a doctor and a scientist. Until modern scientific materialism became the secular religion of our time, and rigorous separation of fields of study were imposed on students and professionals alike, there was no clear distinction between medicine and astrology nor between magic and science.

Seventeenth-century astrologers kept complicated charts in which they reckoned that each disease was caused by a plant; they believed the illness could be cured either by use of herbs belonging to an opposite sign or by sympathy with the herb of the same sign. This "sympathetic magic" form of medicine was practiced in various cultures around the world that have a long-standing tradition of herbal medicine as being closely intertwined with spiritual factors. Thus, plants have for centuries been used in conjunction with astrology and magic to heal, purify, and strengthen the body, and the mind and emotions as well (for these early peoples did not differentiate among them as we do today).

It was believed that plants respond to our thoughts and feelings and that this innate spirit-energy possessed by plants is both the healer and the medicine, which makes herbs sympathetic to our bodies, thus making us sensitive to their healing capacities. Thus, herbal medicine was believed to treat not only the specific complaint but also the entire person, both physical and spiritual.

One quality that both attracted and repelled humans in regard to herbs was their *smell*. Sweet-smelling herbs were valued for many uses, from freshening the stale air of unventilated dwellings to perfuming the body; the strong-smelling herbs could repel biting insects by being rubbed on the skin or scattered on the floor. An example is lavender, which most of us know as the favored scent of talcum-powdered older ladies. It is common knowledge that during Victorian times all properly run homes had linen closets with dried lavender leaves sprinkled between the sheets and blankets stored in them. What is *not* generally known, however, is that lavender is a powerful insecticide. Although it perfumed the linens with a lovely scent, its primary purpose was to kill bedbugs, thus preventing them from biting sleeping humans.

Early herbal use is also intimately connected to cookery, and not just for flavoring purposes. Such strong-smelling herbs as rosemary, thyme, dill, and sage were used to mask the odor of spoiling meat and thus make it edible. To our herb-conscious ancestors, before the days of refrigeration, flavoring of their food was secondary to preserving it.

Probably by accident, early humans learned that certain herbs and spices acted not only to cover up the awful smell of rotting meat, but also to actually keep it fresh longer. Thus was instituted the practice of wrapping fresh-killed and dressed meat in layers of aromatic herbs such as wild mint, sage, basil, and the like.

The Era of Trial and Error

There is no doubt that for much of human history no clear division between the use of plants for food and for medicine was made. For example, wild vegetables—an essential component in all subsistence diets—provided vitamins, minerals, and trace elements. Clearly, people didn't *know* this or have these terms available in their language, but they did know that eating these wild plants kept them healthy or, if they fell sick, helped them get well.

The earliest archaeological evidence we have of prehistoric nutrition comes from excavations in western England and Switzerland, in Neolithic-like villages. These sites have shown that our ancestors enjoyed a remarkably varied assortment of foodstuffs taken from wild nature. Archaeologists discovered remains of mustard, wild rose, bramble, strawberry, crab apple, and a spinach-like weed called orache when they investigated these sites. All of these plants were nutritious foods, and many of them have since become a part of the herbalist's repertoire.

Herbal medicine has always been involved with long-term health and nutrition in an attempt not only to heal but also to prevent illness in the first place. And herbalists have always preferred

WHAT IS FOLK MEDICINE?

According to C. Norman Shealy, M.D., Ph.D., in *The Illustrated Encyclopedia of Natural Remedies,* the term *folk medicine* refers to the traditional beliefs, practices, and materials that people use to maintain health and cope with disease outside of an organized relationship with academic, professionally recognized, and established medical systems and treatments.

The beliefs and practices that make up a system of folk medicine are very closely related to the history, traditions, and life of a recognizable social group. Many people practice folk medicine today, generally working in an environment in which they share the belief system of their patients, and their approach to maintaining health and treating disease.

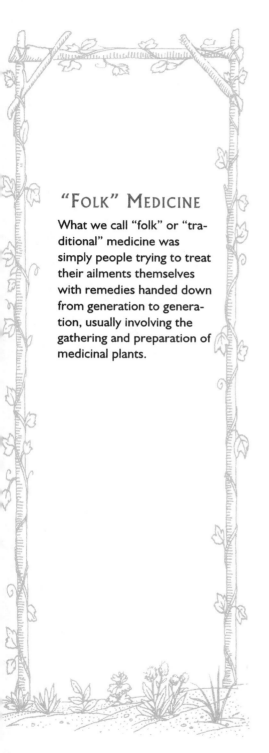

"FOLK" MEDICINE

What we call "folk" or "traditional" medicine was simply people trying to treat their ailments themselves with remedies handed down from generation to generation, usually involving the gathering and preparation of medicinal plants.

the fresh, whole, wild plants for their remedies and potions, knowing instinctively that the wild variety is richer in nutrients than any cultivated plant. (Today, of course, we have full knowledge of the nutrient deficiency of our vegetable food supply, grown as it most often is on poor soil that has been depleted by over-planting and by the soil-destroying methods of agribusiness.)

Thus, food and medicine were complexly intertwined. Much of the discovery of the healing properties of herbs may have occurred accidentally, as when strong-flavored herbs such as hyssop and rosemary, used to preserve foods, were found to have antiseptic or antibacterial action that could be used to treat human ills as well as to keep food from spoiling.

In other cases (such as the famous one of bread mold being the precursor of penicillin), substances or plants were discovered to have healing properties in different forms, such as when dried, ground, chopped, fermented, or otherwise prepared.

Clearly, the majority were discovered by trial and error. Those with quick and dramatic effects—such as purgatives like buckthorn and narcotic-like plants like henbane, which is an excellent painkiller—must have shown their qualities early on. No one knows, of course, just who chewed or brewed the first herbal plants, thus discovering their effects on the human system. What we do know is that in the pre-scientific age, plants were regarded with considerable reverence, even awe. Not only did they have recognizable and predictable effects, but they could appear out of the ground, apparently from nowhere, depending on the season of the year. The secrets of their propagation and growth were beyond human understanding until agricultural communities began to replace nomadic and hunting cultures.

In these communities, the women were the planters, cultivators, gatherers, and harvesters, and thus the primary source of herbal and plant knowledge. Although most medical histories chronicle great deeds and discoveries by men—from Hippocrates, the "father of medicine," to the Greek physician Galen, c.200 C.E., from Paracelsus, in the 16th century, to Alexander Fleming (who discovered penicillin) and Pasteur (who gave us, among other things, pasteurization)—the primary healers have always been women herbalists, who took care of their villagers and who sometimes had reputations that brought patients to them from far and wide. They were also midwives and the earliest pediatricians, not only the persons responsible for the health of pregnant women and successful delivery of their babies but also the persons to whom women turned when their children were ill.

This multitude of women healers have gone by a myriad of names, some of them not complimentary. They have been called wise women, green women, midwives, old wives, nurses, nuns, or anchorites, and—of course—witches.

In the more recent past, herbal and traditional remedies were popular both because they worked and because the people had little other choice. Few could afford to visit a physician, if one was even available. Many lived in small villages or on remote farms, and so a commonsense attitude toward treating the ailments of everyday colds, coughs, infant colic, digestive problems, and the like developed from necessity.

The "natural medicine" practiced was not only first aid for common and minor illnesses, it was also preventative. Some of the most common herbs to be found in the ordinary larder helped to protect against many illnesses, whether or not the people knew specifically how they worked. Onions, garlic, chamomile, mint, sage, thyme, rosemary—all were preventatives, along with a host of others too numerous to name. Although home remedies were a product of necessity, they demonstrably worked. And side effects were few. By incorporating such herbs into their diets, as well as making medicinal use of them, people helped their own health and immune systems to ward off serious disease. The average cottage garden was designed to provide medicinal plants as well as kitchen vegetables and flowers that were not only beautiful but also often had curative properties.

England's Herbal Hero

The advent of the printing press in the 1450s gave herbalism a great boost. The printer William Caxton printed dozens of medical manuals that received wide distribution as the populace was becoming more educated and literate.

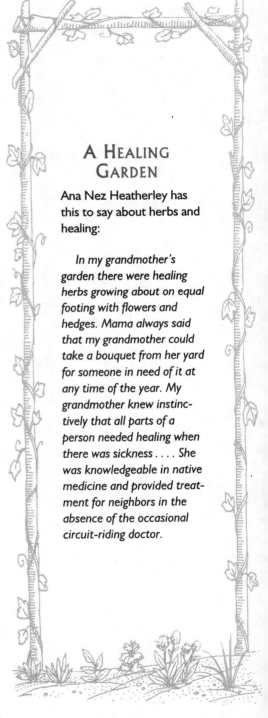

A HEALING GARDEN

Ana Nez Heatherley has this to say about herbs and healing:

In my grandmother's garden there were healing herbs growing about on equal footing with flowers and hedges. Mama always said that my grandmother could take a bouquet from her yard for someone in need of it at any time of the year. My grandmother knew instinctively that all parts of a person needed healing when there was sickness . . . . She was knowledgeable in native medicine and provided treatment for neighbors in the absence of the occasional circuit-riding doctor.

Into this new atmosphere there stepped an eccentric figure often called "The Herbal Robin Hood." Nicholas Culpeper was his name. Among his many accomplishments, he translated the entire physicians' pharmacopoeia, *The English Physician and Complete Herbals* and published it in 1653. It is still in print today, and more than a hundred editions of it have been issued, a record surpassed only by the Bible and the works of Shakespeare.

Yet Culpeper was, in his lifetime, reviled by the powerful Royal College of Physicians for what was then his daring act of translating their learned *Pharmacopoeia* from the classic Latin into "vulgar" English.

Born in 1616, in Surrey, England, Nicholas Culpeper was of aristocratic origins—his family could trace its history back to the time of King John, and they owned vast tracts in the south of England. Nicolas's father was a clergyman, who died 13 days before his son was born, causing his mother to move near her own family. There, he came under the influence of his maternal grandfather—also a clergyman—and learned Greek and Latin. Though his family had planned for him to enter the clergy, he managed to get sent off to Cambridge. There, he distinguished himself in the study of classics and was recognized as a brilliant young scholar with much promise.

An affair of the heart changed his academic career radically. Having fallen passionately in love with a rich young woman who was killed on her way to their wedding when lightning struck her coach, he abruptly left Cambridge, forfeiting the inheritance he could have had from his grandfather. He apprenticed himself to an apothecary at Bishopgate in order to take up the serious study of herbal medicines and of astrology. In 1640, he married a young girl, Alice Field, and, with her dowry, set up his own apothecary practice in Red Lion Street, Spitalfields, in London's East End, where he devoted himself to providing medicines and medical advice to the poor of London.

He dedicated himself to collecting and recording as much information as he could garner about the uses of medicinal plants native to England, gathering much of this information from the local "herb women" who sold local herbs to the London apothecaries for their use in filling the prescriptions detailed by the physicians in the *London Pharmacopoeia*. This Latin tome was the "secret handbook" of the physicians and contained all their recipes for combining herbs for various medical treatments.

During the English Civil War, which set Oliver Cromwell and his Puritan Parliament against King Charles I, Culpeper went further against his class by choosing to side with Cromwell. He was thus, or so it seems, accused of witchcraft. In addition, always unorthodox, the aristocrat-turned-herbalist had outraged the entire London medical establishment by having the bold nerve to render the highly secret *Pharmacopoeia Londinensis* into English, giving it the title of *The London Dispensatory and Physical Directory*.

As a Puritan and anti-monarchist, Culpeper bitterly resented the snobbery of the monarchist College of Physicians who basically ignored the medical needs of the poor and largely Puritan classes. His solution was as simple as Robin Hood's: to take from the rich and give to the poor. His motives were noble, too: he wanted to expose the unnecessarily secret and, therefore, exclusive practices of the physicians' guild in order to make herbal medicines available to poor people unable to pay the physicians' exorbitant fees, with which they milked the rich.

This act of derring-do earned Culpeper the undying hatred of the Royal College of Physicians, but it also endeared him to the common people—apothecaries, midwives, and the poor—for giving them ready access to the formerly closely held professional medical information. Those who were illiterate in Latin had their first glimpse at the thousands of formulae that constituted what was, in the 17th century, England's medical state of the art.

Undaunted by the contemporary medical establishment's enmity, Culpeper went on to publish in 1651 the first English textbook on midwifery and child care, *The English Midwife*, emphasizing the necessity of cleanliness (at a time when surgeons regularly went from the autopsy room to deliver babies without washing their hands) and proper nutrition for the mother-to-be and

THE ARABIC INFLUENCE

Prior to the resurgence of herbal medicine in England in the 1700s, great medical advances had been introduced by the Arabs, who, through their occupation of Spain, had brought both alchemy and the pharmacy into Western medicine. They introduced new ointments, elixirs, pills, tinctures, suppositories, purgatives, cathartics, and inhalations. It was through their influence that apothecaries burgeoned in England from the 12th century on. But it was not until the mid-16th century that Paracelsus, today considered the founder of chemical pharmacology, taught that alchemy and chemistry could be combined to unlock the secrets of Nature's healing herbs and plants.

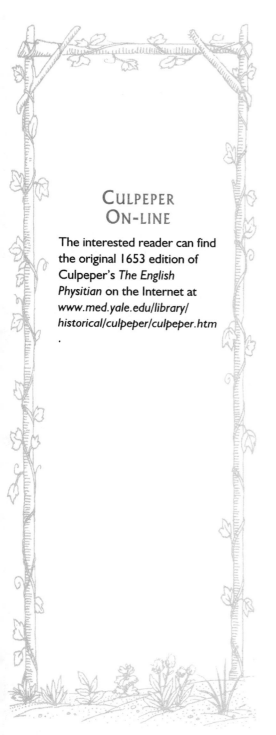

CULPEPER
ON-LINE

The interested reader can find the original 1653 edition of Culpeper's *The English Physitian* on the Internet at *www.med.yale.edu/library/historical/culpeper/culpeper.htm*
.

the newborn. The book provided herbal remedies for the common problems associated with pregnancy and childbirth.

And in the same year, he published *Judgement of Disease,* a diagnostic manual designed to teach ordinary people how to understand their bodies and their ills.

After bringing out the famous *Complete Herbal and English Physician* in 1652, Nicholas Culpeper himself became ill and died in 1654. Some say the cause was tuberculosis, but modern psychology might point to overwork, stress, and rejection by his peers as important factors. Fortunately, Culpeper had tutored his young wife in the skills and lore of herbal medicine, and she continued to publish his books.

Writing about Culpeper, Susan Wittig Albert, Ph.D., comments that it isn't difficult to understand why the College of Physicians was made apoplectic by Culpeper's publication of their tightly held secrets. She points out that they were afraid of him with good reason, saying that Nicholas Culpeper was "smart, outspoken, and self-assured, ready to take on the medical establishment and to point out that the emperor had no clothes. He was vehement in his rejection of the expensive imported exotic plants that the College preferred, pointing out that there were plenty of herbs free for the picking in field and heath that would do just as well."

Seen in the context of his own time and political situation, it is clear that Culpeper made a valuable contribution to our knowledge of the history of the medicinal plants he understood so well—far better than anyone else of his day. He taught that it is important for people to learn how their bodies function and have information about the readily available herbal remedies they could utilize for various ailments, and he gave instructions for the making and use of these simple, natural healers.

In the end, it was probably Culpeper's devotion to astrology that ruined him as much as anything else. In choosing to use the astrological model to explain the relationships between the plants and the planets, he came up against the new Enlightenment philosophies that declared reason was all, and in rejecting astrological concepts as a valid component of medical treatment, he threw out the baby with the bathwater, as the saying goes.

CULPEPER'S HERBS

In Culpeper's day, there were only five known planets: Mercury, Venus, Mars, Jupiter, and Saturn (in addition to the sun and the moon, which are called "lights," not planets). He arranged herbs according to their relationships with the planets and zodiacal signs. Following are some of the most familiar:

SUN—
ZODIACAL SIGN
OF LEO
Chamomile
Eyebright
St. John's wort
Lovage
Marigold (calendula)
Peony
Rosemary
Rue
Saffron

MOON—
ZODIACAL SIGN
OF CANCER
Cabbage
Columbine
Watercress
Ivy
Lettuce
Moonwort
Poppy
Purslane
White roses
Willow

MERCURY—
ZODIACAL SIGN
OF GEMINI
AND VIRGO
Dill
Fern
Fennel
Horehound
Lavender
Licorice
Maidenhair
Sweet marjoram
Parsley
Southernwood

VENUS—
ZODIACAL SIGN
OF TAURUS
AND LIBRA
Lady's bedstraw
Chickweed
Cowslips
Daisies
Elder
Goldenrod
Lady's mantle
Mint
Plantain
Sorrel

Strawberries
Tansy
Violet
Yarrow

MARS—
ZODIACAL SIGN
OF ARIES
AND SCORPIO
Basil
Garlic
Hawthorn
Hops
Mustard
Onions
Radish
Horseradish
Rhubarb
Thistle
Tobacco
Wormwood

JUPITER—
ZODIACAL SIGN
OF SAGITTARIUS
AND PISCES
Agrimony
Bay
Bilberry

Borage
Costmary
Dandelion
Dock
Hyssop
Liverwort
Red roses
Sage

SATURN—
ZODIACAL SIGN
OF CAPRICORN
AND AQUARIUS
Cleavers
Comfrey
Dodder
Goutwort
Hemlock
Hemp
Henbane
Horsetail
Mullein
Nightshade

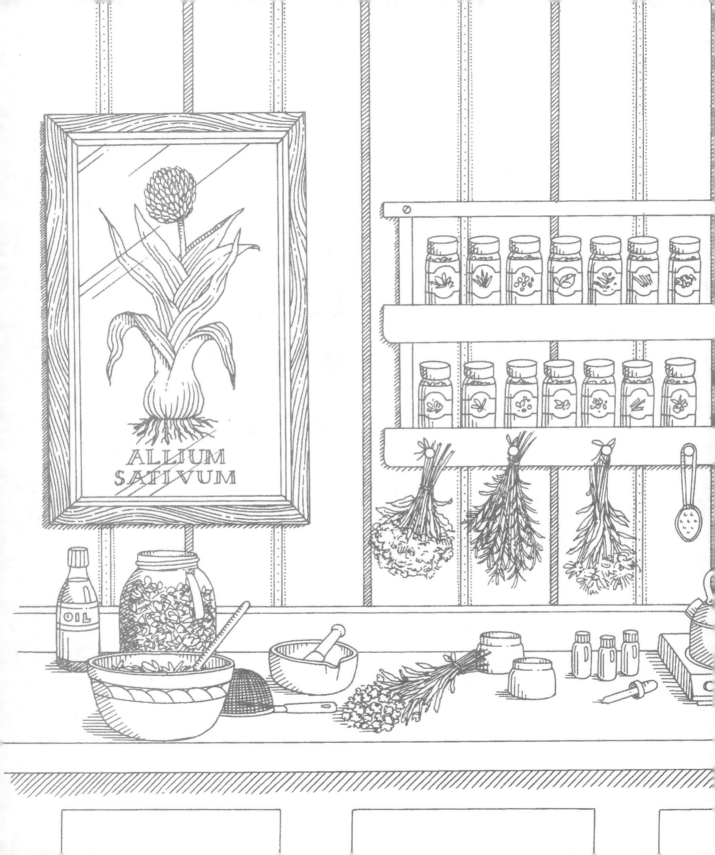

ALLIUM
SATIVUM

OIL

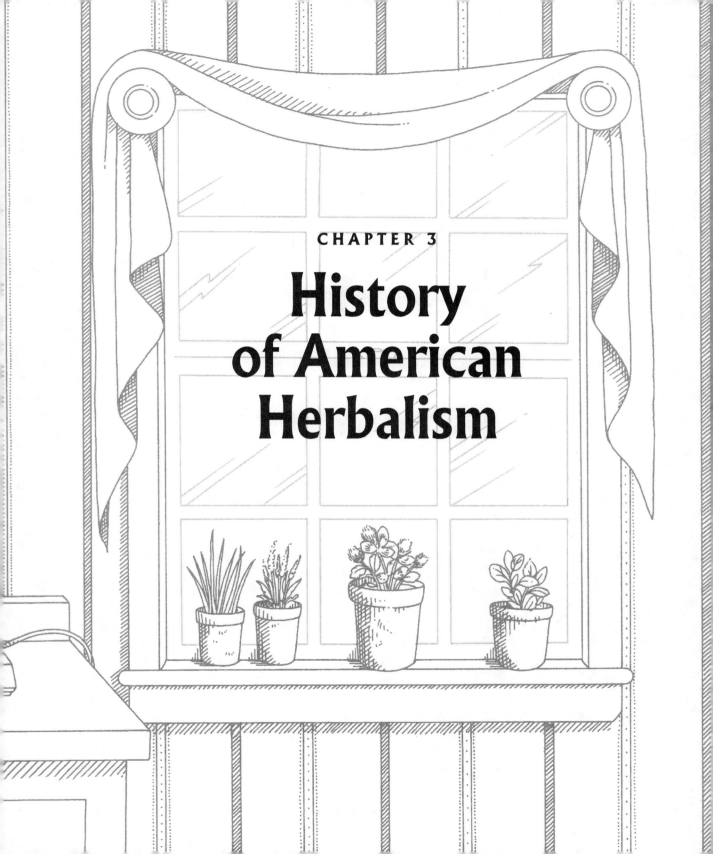

CHAPTER 3

History of American Herbalism

There is nothing in the most advanced contemporary medicine whose embryo cannot be found in the medicine of the past.

—MAXIMILLEN E.P. LITTRÉ

The first European settlers arriving in North America brought with them the familiar healing plants from home: heartsease and plantain. However, they encountered health problems that they had never expected when they landed on these shores and began to make settlements—problems their native plants alone could not cure. Although the Europeans who came to the New World mostly looked upon the Native Americans as ignorant savages, there was one important exception: their knowledge of plants, not only which ones to grow and how to plant them but also how to use them for health and healing.

Only too familiar with plagues, pestilence, ill health, poor medical care, and a host of other ills back home, the colonists and explorers who came to these shores were eager to learn what they could from the superbly healthy Indians, who had fine, strong physiques, physical stamina, and good teeth, and who were willing to share their incomparable knowledge of the indigenous plants with the settlers, who out of necessity became apt students of native herbal medicine. The stiff-necked Puritan Cotton Mather wrote that the Indian healers produced "many cures that are truly stupendous." And the founder of Methodism, John Wesley, upon visiting America in the 1730s, wrote in amazement that the Indians had "exceedingly few" diseases, noting that their medicinal herbal treatments were "quick and generally infallible."

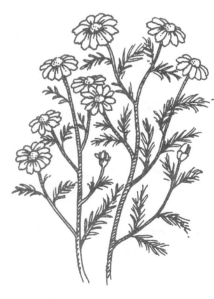

The Indians were exceptionally gifted at the treatment of wounds, and they earned the admiration of the U.S. Army, whose members were astonished by the effectiveness of Indian treatments for battle and other wounds. As a result, early American physicians often gave themselves over to apprenticeship with Indian "medicine men" healers, who introduced the white settlers to many valuable herbs such as black and blue cohosh, black haw, boneset (a particularly welcome gift during a serious flu epidemic), cascara sagrada, echinacea, chaparral, goldenseal, lobelia, Oregon grape, sarsaparilla, slippery elm, wild cherry, and witch hazel—to name just a few.

Despite this generosity, American University-trained doctors looked down their noses at this "savage" medicine. The noted Philadelphia doctor and a signer of the Declaration of Independence, Benjamin Rush, wrote: "We have no discoveries in the *materia medica* . . . from the Indians. It would be a reproach to our schools of physic if modern physicians were not more successful than Indians."

Rush was proved wrong on more than one occasion. American colonists planted both medicinal and culinary herbs in their well-tended gardens. Thomas Jefferson, an ardent gardener, grew 26 herbs at Monticello in his "kitchen garden."

New World Botanic Medicine

The first American herbalist of note was Samuel Thomson (1760–1843), who was born in Alstead, New Hampshire. Thomson studied with Indian healers and, as a child, had learned from a local midwife, the Widow Benton, a "root and herb" doctor who combined Native American skills with the traditional role of "herb woman" or "herb wife" (another term for midwife). The turning point for Thomson came in 1800, or thereabouts, when his daughter became seriously ill. Extremely worried about her worsening condition, he called in a regular physician who pronounced her "incurable." At this point, Thomson turned to his own knowledge of Indian healing and herbal treatments and cured her himself using the Indian "sweat lodge" form of detoxification and herbs he prepared.

Inspired by his unexpected success, Thomson began calling himself "doctor" and treating patients by his unorthodox methods. He had come to detest the methods of the doctors of his day—bleeding was one of the most popular (and ineffective as well as debilitating) "treatments," used for just about anything. Other doubtful treatments included extremely strong purgatives and the use of mercury, which we know today is poisonous.

These so-called "heroic" methods were, unfortunately, often deadly rather than curative. For example, in 1799 the illustrious father of our country, George Washington, developed flu-like symptoms—a sore throat, fever, and chills. Washington was elderly but

THE ROLE OF ONIONS IN HISTORY

The idea of having a salad with every dinner is a twentieth-century innovation.

However, many of the foods we use in salads were a part of the diet of our great-grandparents. Those dishes consisted of lettuce, onions, and radishes in late spring; coleslaw during the summer; endive, turnip slaw, and celery during crisp autumn days; and dandelion and watercress in early spring . . . . One old writing suggests that, "At this season of the year (spring) too much cannot be said in favor of onions. Whether raw or cooked they are especially good, both medicinally and as a skin beautifier."

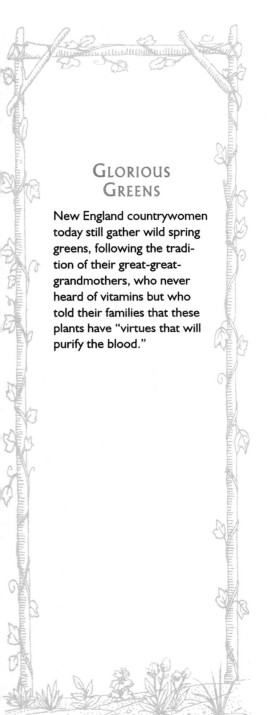

GLORIOUS GREENS

New England countrywomen today still gather wild spring greens, following the tradition of their great-great-grandmothers, who never heard of vitamins but who told their families that these plants have "virtues that will purify the blood."

in generally good health. Probably he had some minor infection that would have been cured by the same simple means we use today—rest, abundant hot liquids, mild herbal antibiotics like garlic and onion, and time to allow his body to heal itself. But this was not to be.

His physician first bled him of 4 pints of blood—the human body contains only 8 pints of blood altogether!—and then dosed him with mercury and strong laxatives. Anemic and weakened by these "heroic" medical measures, in 24 hours he was dead.

Similar scenarios were typical, and this outraged Samuel Thomson. He went on to develop his own medical system, which he called "physiomedicalism," based on what he had learned of European herbalism from the midwives who brought their knowledge to these shores and on what he had learned from his Indian healer tutors. He favored hot mineral baths and sweat lodges as well as various herbal remedies that he concocted himself.

One of the herbs he particularly favored was lobelia, which, if given in large doses, can cause vomiting. As a result of administering what was alleged to be a fatal amount of lobelia, he was accused of murder in 1809. But he was acquitted, due to lack of evidence that lobelia is poisonous. Nonetheless, his New Hampshire rivals, the regular physicians, conspired to drum him out of their state, prevailing on the New Hampshire legislature to name him as a person forbidden to practice medicine.

Undaunted by this concerted action against him and his methods, he moved to Ohio, setting up his practice there.

He patented Thomson's Improved System of Botanic Practice of Medicine, a combination of handbooks and patent remedies that became immensely popular nationwide early in the 19th century. At one time, as word of his treatments spread, he claimed three million adherents to his system, which may have been an exaggeration, but there was no doubt that Thomson's herbalism was taken up with enthusiasm by large numbers of people everywhere. He died in 1843, after which his methods waned in popularity.

After Thomson's death, a few physicians, calling themselves "naturopaths," continued using physiomedical methods, and the herb-and-bath system of treatment, one of these being Dr. John Kellogg of Battle Creek, Michigan. In an attempt to create the perfect health food, Kellogg inadvertently founded the first cereal manufacturer. Kellogg believed grains to be the most healthful of foods and was a strict vegetarian. After much experimentation, he accidentally stumbled on a method of "rolling" grains into flakes—giving us the now ubiquitous cornflake. Kellogg had many adherents to his health system, but eventually it, too, faded away, to be replaced by homeopathy and what was called "eclectic herbalism."

America's Herbal Scientists

Surprisingly, considering the routine bleeding, purgation, and use of mercury by "regular" physicians, most medicines of the 19th century were herbal—that is, based on botanicals. In 1820, the *United States Pharmacopoeia's* list of treatments was $2/3$ botanical, and in 1880 the percentage was almost $3/4$.

Following the lead of Thomson's physiomedicalism, during the 1820s an eclectic combination of practitioners—Thomsonians, herbalists trained by Native Americans, and "regular" doctors who had become disillusioned with what they saw their colleagues doing—gathered together and formed an organization they called the Reformed Medical Society for the purpose of promoting alternative methods in opposition to the heroic ones commonly practiced. Largely, they used herbal remedies. Then, in 1830, led by Dr. Wooster Beech, the group founded a medical school to teach their methods.

As the East Coast cities were a bastion of what the reformers called "regular medicine," meaning heroic, they located their school near Columbus, Ohio, which at that time was still frontier territory and therefore much more open minded than the established eastern part of the country. Settling on the Mississippi River, they decided to call their method *eclectic* because it was a combi-

THE CORN IS GREEN

The Native American word for *corn* meant "our life," or "our mother," or "she who sustains us." This attitude toward plants extended to all things that grew from the earth that sustained life for the Indians, especially the medicinal plants, which they treated with reverence and incorporated into their religious tradition, out of which grew the songs, dances, ceremonials, and worship they believed sustained the principle of life—of survival itself. The burning of sage as a purifying smoke is an example of an herb's ceremonial use.

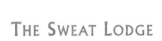

The Sweat Lodge

The "sweat lodge" was a sauna-like structure filled with hot coals that heated the air to a high temperature. Its purpose was to induce copious perspiration in the sick person in order to rid the body of toxins and bacteria.

Magical Medicine

Native American herbalism was shamanistic, centering on the "medicine man," who, through the use of drums, rattles, and the smoking of mixtures of tobacco or peyote, entered a trancelike state that enabled him to "spirit-travel" in order to seek out the soul of the sick person, rescue it, and thus heal the illness.

nation of European, Asian, Native American, and African slave herbalism. Thus they became known as Eclectics.

So progressive-minded were they that when they moved their Eclectic Medical Institute to Cincinnati in 1845, they admitted women as students. These were women who were already followers of Thomsonian herbalism who wanted more training in their profession. Unfortunately, however—as a precursor to the practice of excluding women from medical schools in the 20th century—in 1877 the Eclectics barred women students. According to the Eclectic historian, Henry Felter, they "yielded to the prejudices of the profession."

The Eclectics considered themselves to be "scientific herbalists," and as such they performed experiments with herbs and analyzed their chemical components, extracting their active constituents. Their findings were published in the scientific journals of the period and were well received by the pharmaceutical industry.

After the decline of Eclecticism, herbal healing experienced a Dark Age, which lasted until the 1960s when the "hippie" movement revitalized interest in herbal medicine. Establishment medical schools had ignored herbs (just as they ignored nutrition in general), and the influx of new pharmaceutical drugs drove herbal remedies out of the nation's pharmacies. Even the ever-popular culinary herbs suffered a decline, being replaced by manufactured mixtures that often contained synthetic ingredients, artificial flavorings, and the now notorious MSG flavor enhancer.

However, like magic and truth, herbal healing didn't really die—it just went underground, literally, until the new revolutionaries called hippies started the "back to the land" movement. These new renegades of society, despising the Establishment (as they dubbed all that was stridently orthodox), began to grow their own herbs (yes, including the outlawed marijuana, which has since been proven to have medicinal value). As usual, folk medicine continued to be practiced by women, who, having been excluded from the all-male medical establishment, had always kept the tradition alive. Some men, too, joined their forces to grow and gather herbs and use and prescribe them as the classic herbal manuals recommended.

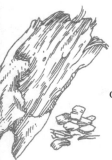

These diehards kept the tradition alive by following the lead of Dr. Benedict Lust, the father of modern naturopathy, who had come to the United States from Germany in 1895 and opened the nation's first health food store. Dr. Lust went on to establish sanitariums in New Jersey and Florida similar to the German *kur-bad*, literally translated as "cure bath," where herbal baths and herbal infusions taken internally played an important part in the cure.

During the 19th century, the royal and the elite frequented such tony sites as Baden-Baden and Weisbaden, the capital of Bavarian royalty. Lesser folk could also take advantage of one of a multitude of these health centers. Many were run by the government, which strongly believed in preventative health measures and in rejuvenation through herbal tonics and baths. Whole towns were given over to state-sponsored *kur-bads*. Rules for peace and quiet were strictly enforced, and the mineral waters peculiar to each were carefully protected by the government. These towns were famous for their mineral waters, which were carefully analyzed and their components publicly listed. Today in Germany, any town with the word *bad* in it has a *kur–bad*. One such town is Bad Bruckenau, founded by King Ludwig of Bavaria.

People went to "take the waters," both internally for rejuvenation and healing and externally by immersion. Dr. Lust based his sanitariums on the same principles that were the basis of the German *bad*—healing herbal baths, wraps, and herbal medicines. His nephew, John Lust, wrote about his uncle's work in *The Herb Book*.

The Hippie Herbal Revolution

Unlike in Britain, says California herbalist Amanda McQuare Crawford, "herbal medicine in the U.S. is a do-it-yourself business. This is partly because there simply hasn't been the training . . . . But it's also partly because America has a long tradition dating back to pioneer times of sturdy self-sufficiency in herbal medicine. Out on the frontiers of civilization there weren't any practitioners, every ranch housewife had to be her own herbal expert. There

THOMSON'S "VITAL FORCE" PHILOSOPHY

Central to the physiomedical system was the notion that it is possible to strengthen the body's "vital force" by keeping the physical body's tissues in balance with the person's nervous state. The key therapeutic treatment involved relaxing or tightening tissues while either sedating or stimulating the nervous system. Herbs classified as relaxing or astringent, stimulating or sedating, were prescribed for this purpose.

HERB-BASED DRUGS

Today, almost all drugs and over-the-counter remedies are in some way based on herbalism. Apparently, drug companies are always attempting to duplicate Nature's wisdom! Many of these preparations are synthetic compounds of naturally occurring substances.

has never been a real medicalisation of herbal medicine: most of the books are aimed at this amateur market to a degree which would be unthinkable in England."

And, says Barbara Griggs, "the recent history of phytotherapy in the United States is one of legal suppression that almost succeeded in wiping the collective memory clean."

But there was a strong desire sweeping the land that was exemplified by the so-called hippie back-to-the-land movement, itself an echo of those pioneering times of self-sufficiency. Michael Tierra, one of America's best known herbalists today and the author of the bestseller *The Way of Herbs*, was one of those latter-day pioneers. He says:

> *I didn't have any background in herbal medicine. It grew out of my personal experience as an artist, a musician, and a beatnik in the late '50s and early '60s. There was a whole crowd of us in Haight Asbury in San Francisco: we were in search of an alternative lifestyle, and we experimented with herbs to try and solve our health problems.*
>
> *A company of us bought some wilderness land in the North California Mountains, and started a community there—we called it Black Bear Ranch.*

Michael's ranch had no running water and no electricity, and its communal goal was self-sufficiency. They grew their own food and watched their children being born and raised. Michael combed the bookshops for information on herbalism, finding little information. He found Maud Grieve's *Modern Herbal*, a classic which had been published in London in 1931; Jethro Kloss's *Back to Eden*, which became the hippie herbal bible; and a 1918 paperback by Joseph E. Meyer called simply *The Herbalist*, which contained information on Native American use of herbs but included few details. Says Tierra, "I was just totally attracted and amazed by all the plants around me—they just grabbed me by the seat of my pants, and I knew I wanted to know more."

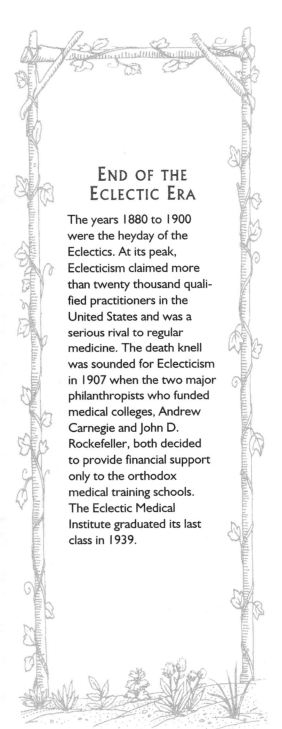

END OF THE ECLECTIC ERA

The years 1880 to 1900 were the heyday of the Eclectics. At its peak, Eclecticism claimed more than twenty thousand qualified practitioners in the United States and was a serious rival to regular medicine. The death knell was sounded for Eclecticism in 1907 when the two major philanthropists who funded medical colleges, Andrew Carnegie and John D. Rockefeller, both decided to provide financial support only to the orthodox medical training schools. The Eclectic Medical Institute graduated its last class in 1939.

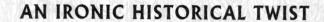

AN IRONIC HISTORICAL TWIST

In his search for an easily digestible food to serve to the illustrious patrons of his Battle Creek Sanitarium, Dr. Kellogg invented toasted grain flakes in 1894, establishing the Battle Creek Toasted Corn Flake Company in 1906. However, Kellogg was not motivated solely by profit; he was a philanthropist who, during the Great Depression, added an extra shift at the factory, paying workers more for fewer hours. Ten years ago, Kellogg's share of the American cereal market was 42 percent, but that share has dropped to 32 percent.

U.S. News and World Report's August 30, 1999, issue reported that Joseph Stewart, Kellogg's senior vice president for corporate affairs, announced the closing of the historic South Plant, calling it "an inefficient relic of a bygone era." Kellogg will eliminate 550 jobs with the closing, which is projected to save them up to $45 million a year as they shift operations to the newer North Plant and to other manufacturing sites around the world.

Comments *U.S. News and World Report*: A sound strategy, perhaps, but not one that cornflake creator, Dr. J. H. Kellogg . . . would have approved. An eccentric advocate of "biological eating," [Dr. Kellogg] insisted on restricting sales to patients. "I am not after the business, I am after the reform," he said.

HERBS BY THE TON

In 1959, the United States imported 500,000 tons of the herb fennel; 467,000 tons of oregano, and 5 million tons of red pepper. By 1986, these figures had risen to 5 million tons of fennel, 12 million tons of oregano, and 14 million tons of red pepper.

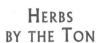

MILKWEED WARNING

All milkweeds are poisonous if taken in large amounts. The more narrow-leafed plants are the most toxic. Herbalists today do not recommend taking milkweed internally.

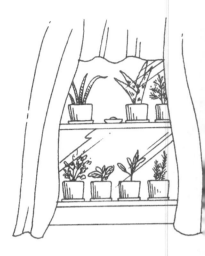

Finally he went to the original source, the Native Americans themselves, to begin his education. He also became a pupil of a controversial figure, Dr. John Christopher, who followed Samuel Thomson's precepts of herbal healing. As a result of his and others' efforts, by the 1960s, many Americans had experienced a change of attitude about their health and healing, deciding to invest their means in prevention instead of "cure" after the fact. Interestingly, one of the reasons herbs were revived was the tremendous press coverage warning about overuse of salt, which research had linked to high blood pressure, heart disease, and stroke.

A salt-loving nation that gobbled down salty potato chips, salted peanuts, and a variety of other heavily salted snacks suddenly became conscious of the seemingly innocuous substance they ingested so freely. Voila! Herbs and spices had a renaissance in the home kitchens of America—and even Chinese restaurants, once heavy users of MSG, proclaimed on their menus, "No MSG Used."

Not only were imports rising to an astronomical degree in response to the demand, but domestic production became big business as well. Individuals began growing herbs on their windowsills and farmers took to sowing herbs in their fields for mass production, with the result that an astounding number of herbal products now line the shelves of supermarkets, as well as those of health food stores, and mail-order catalogs specializing in herbs and herbal products abound.

According to Michael Castleman, in his book *The Healing Herbs*, published in 1991, authoritative estimates of retail sales of healing herbs, kitchen spices, herb books, herbal beverage teas, and herbal cosmetics and personal care products now top $3 billion annually, and the boom continues unabated.

Castleman also reports that (as his book went to press) United States herbalists, led by the American Botanical Council (ABC) in Austin, Texas, hoped to persuade the FDA to create a drug category for Folklore Medicine. However, the executive director of ABC, Mark Blumenthal, told Castleman that the FDA has given no indication that it will treat age-old herbal remedies differently from new pharmaceuticals. This is unfortunate, but because healing herbs cannot be patented, there is little to no incentive for research to either prove or disprove their traditional usage and/or effectiveness. The sad fact is that the pharmaceutical companies that market drugs and make fortunes from them are more concerned with showing a profit for their shareholders than promoting the health of the general populace. They isolate the active constituents of healing herbs and then fiddle around with them to produce something chemically unique so that they can then patent drugs they develop from these "new" chemicals. As a result of this, few physicians—let alone patients—realize that many of the drugs they prescribe have herbal origins.

Says Barbara Griggs in *The Green Pharmacy*:

When we talk of "chemical" as opposed to "natural" medicine, therefore, we are actually talking nonsense: all medicine, from the greenest witch-doctor brew to the most potent substance concocted in a pharmaceutical laboratory is composed of "chemicals." The difference is in the way they are produced; and in the way they are packaged.

But a growing body of perfectly respectable scientific research suggests that there may, after all, be plenty more to be said, and that we are only at the beginning of a new knowledge of what plants and men and life itself are about, and how intricately man and plant interrelate.

In the light of the evidence—whether there actually is a difference between the chemical components of a living plant and man-made chemicals derived from that plant—it would seem to be simple common sense to recognize that the human body itself acts as if there indeed is a difference. Herbal medicines have few

THE FOXY FOXGLOVE

An English physician, William Withering, was treating a patient suffering from severe dropsy caused by heart failure. The patient's relatives administered an herbal concoction brewed from an old family recipe, and the man recovered. Dr. Withering began to experiment with herbs contained in the recipe and identified foxglove as the major component. In 1785, after 10 years of studying foxglove and its side effects, he published a book entitled *Account of the Foxglove and Some of Its Medical Uses*. This study detailed two hundred cases he had treated with the herb successfully and included his extensive research notes.

Further analysis followed and in time the cardiac glycosides digoxin and digitoxin were isolated and extracted, giving us the drug digitalis, which is used to treat heart conditions today.

DAISIES FOR THE LITTLE PEOPLE

The delicate white flowers of fleabane are extremely pretty and have earned them the name "daisies for the Little People," among Native American tribes who have used fleabane flowers. The tiny flowers are dried and made into a sort of snuff, which is used for inflammation of the nasal passages. Several tribes found fleabane useful for kidney problems, including kidney stones, and as a diuretic. Its use could bring on sneezing, and so it was considered good for clearing congestion, and a tea made from the delicate flowers supposedly made headaches go away. The entire plant was used as part of the ritual of the sweat lodge, in which many different herbs and plants were employed, depending on the specific purpose the particular sweat lodge was intended to serve.

or no side effects; but the long list of noxious side effects experienced by those subjected to pharmaceutically extracted derivatives of these plants is in itself eloquent testimony to the validity of the actual, and entire, plant's medicinal value.

And whether supported by modern medicine's claims to be the ultimate authority or not, herbal medicine has an undisputed history of thousands of years of recorded clinical use that has noted their rare side effects. Therefore, reason would suggest that any plant used for medicinal purposes that has a centuries-long reputation behind it as being completely safe as well as effective has legitimately earned that reputation.

The Native American Herbal Tradition

Native American folklore and tradition have played a major role in a five-thousand-year-old history proving the health and healing value of herbs. The Cherokees used ragweed for insect bites and hives; other Native American tribes used it for the treatment of diabetes, pneumonia, nausea, and worms, and as a sedative. They also used the seeds of the giant ragweed as a food source.

Another plant Native Americans used for a multitude of purposes was buttonbush, which is still used among indigenous people who live close to the land. In earlier days, it was used as an astringent; the inner bark was macerated for toothache; and a tea made from the leaf was a diuretic, a treatment for fever, and a means to decrease menstrual flow.

We don't know if Native Americans kept cats as pets or only knew them as wild animals, but they used catnip as a treatment for colds, fevers, headache, and diarrhea, and to bring on menstruation as well as soothe menstrual cramps. In addition, this useful plant was considered a tranquilizer and used to promote restful sleep.

Among the many Native American tribes that used the plant for medicine, the Cherokees specifically favored it to rid the intestines of worms and for general digestive upset, including colic in infants. They diapered their babies with the soft down produced by the cattail plant, which prevented "diaper rash" and could also be used to treat burns. Native Americans taught early settlers to use cattail for food.

HOXSEY'S HERBAL HOAX

One of American herbalism's oddest cases is that of Harry Hoxsey, who, in the middle of the 20th century loudly proclaimed that his herbal formula could cure cancer. Hoxsey, born in Appalachia and a former coal miner there, had no formal education other than a correspondence high school diploma. Nevertheless, he produced what he called the Hoxsey Cancer Formula, which he claimed to have learned from his great-grandfather, who had seen a cancer-ridden horse cured of the disease after eating various herbs.

Beginning in the 1930s, Hoxsey prescribed the family formula and by the 1950s had established a clinic in Dallas that was the world's largest privately owned treatment facility for cancer. It had branches in seventeen states. During the 1930s, he was arrested for fraud more than a hundred times by a Dallas prosecutor who, to his dismay, could not find witnesses against Hoxsey to attest they had been defrauded. Hundreds of his patients came to his defense, saying they had been cured by his formula. Despite this support, Hoxsey had run afoul of the powerful American Medical Association (AMA). Eventually the Food and Drug Administration (FDA) forced the closing of his clinics on the basis that he had violated federal regulations regarding the labeling of drugs (herbs were not on the list of approved cancer treatments).

Ironically, Hoxsey himself died of prostate cancer even though he took his own formula. However, it is still available—though not in the United States. The Bio-Medical Center in Tijuana, Mexico, uses it, and many Americans have traveled there to avail themselves of it. Another irony about Hoxsey's "hoax," as it was alleged to be, is that recent studies of the formula have shown nine of its ten herbal components to have anti-tumor properties. They are barberry, buckthorn, burdock, cascara sagrada, red clover, licorice, poke, prickly ash, and bloodroot.

AN ANTI-WITCHCRAFT HERB

The herb gay feather was used by the peoples indigenous to both the United States and Mexico as a talisman against witchcraft, *mal de ojo* (the evil eye, or evil spells). Its root was cut in half, and one part was carved into a cross that was worn as a protective amulet, especially by small children who were thought to be especially vulnerable.

In addition, the Cherokee used the root for aches and pains in the limbs. Smoke from it was inhaled to stop nosebleed and headache, and blown down a patient's throat for tonsillitis.

Another favorite of the Cherokees was crimson clover, a multiple purpose plant used for coughs and lung conditions such as asthma, bronchitis, and chronic coughing. The Cherokees also made a tea from cocklebur for use as a diuretic, as well as for bladder infections, to stop wounds, and to stop bleeding. Echinacea was used extensively for any number of problems; it was made into a tea or a tincture.

The Navajos were particularly fond of cota, or Navajo tea, which grew in the mountains of New Mexico. It was used as a drink, as well as for its medicinal properties, which are soothing and calming.

A species of rumex called "dock" was popular with various tribes who used a poultice from the plant root to treat wounds. It has a high content of both vitamins A and C. Native Americans who live in Arizona still use it for colds and sore throats.

The Cherokee made an ointment of mallow flowers for sores and poultices for tumors (other tribes used it for arthritis and healing wounds). And mesquite beans provided a major food supply for them; a basic tea made from mesquite stems, leaves, and bark was used both internally and externally.

They had only to follow the beautiful monarch butterfly to find another frequently used herb, milkweed, which was used as a laxative. The Cherokees boiled the seeds in fresh milk to stop diarrhea; other Native Americans used milkweed for treating swellings, fever, and pneumonia.

Native Americans taught settlers to use milkweed as a diuretic, to break a fever, and as an expectorant for respiratory illnesses such as bronchitis and asthma. The root was powdered and made into a paste with water for a skin emollient. It was also used in ceremonials as an emetic for cleansing purposes.

Another favorite ceremonial herb used by Native American Indians for cleansing as well as for the sweat lodge was mint. Inhalation of a hot infusion was believed to improve concentration.

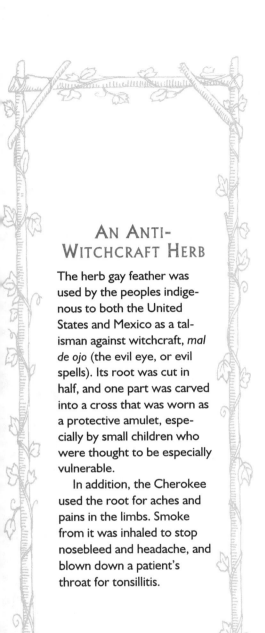

HEALING PLANTS NATIVE TO
NORTH AMERICA

ALGERITA	HOREHOUND	POKE
ALOE	HORSETAIL	PRAIRIE TEA
AMARANTH	INDIGO	PRICKLY POPPY
APACHE-PLUME	JIMSONWEED	PURSLANE
BEE BALM	JUJUBE	QUEEN'S DELIGHT
BRIER	JUNIPER	RATANY
BROOMWEED	LAMB'S-QUARTERS	SAGEBRUSH
CATALPA	LARKSPUR	SAW PALMETTO
CATCLAW	LEMON BALM	SELF-HEAL
CENTURY PLANT	LEMONGRASS	SENNA
CHAPARRAL	LICORICE	SHEPHERD'S PURSE
CHASTE TREE	MAIDENHAIR FERN	SKULLCAP
CHICKWEED	MALLOW	SOAPBERRY
CINQUEFOIL	MESQUITE	SOAPWORT
CLEAVERS	MILKWEED	SPIDERWORT
CLOVER (SWEET)	MINT	STONECROP
DANDELION	MULLEIN	SUMAC
DESERT WILLOW	MUSTARD	TEASEL
DEVIL'S CLAW	NIGHTSHADE	TRUMPET VINE
EVENING PRIMROSE	OLD-MAN'S-BEARD	WATERCRESS
GOAT'S HEAD	PASSIONFLOWER	YARROW
GOLDENROD	PERIWINKLE	YUCCA
HOP TREE	PLANTAIN	

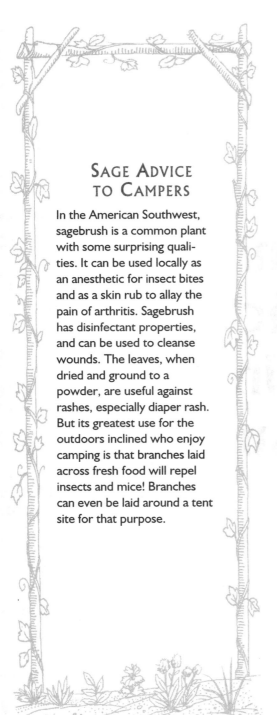

SAGE ADVICE TO CAMPERS

In the American Southwest, sagebrush is a common plant with some surprising qualities. It can be used locally as an anesthetic for insect bites and as a skin rub to allay the pain of arthritis. Sagebrush has disinfectant properties, and can be used to cleanse wounds. The leaves, when dried and ground to a powder, are useful against rashes, especially diaper rash. But its greatest use for the outdoors inclined who enjoy camping is that branches laid across fresh food will repel insects and mice! Branches can even be laid around a tent site for that purpose.

Although we shudder at the thought of "deadly nightshade," we regularly consume its relatives, tomatoes and potatoes. However, several Native American tribes used the plant internally to rid themselves of intestinal parasites and administered it also for fevers, eye problems, and insomnia. And they made salves from it for skin eruptions and sores. They also taught the settlers this process.

The beautiful redbud tree is among the first to signal the arrival of spring. Its lovely pink-red flowers appear before the foliage. Native Americans used redbud flowers to make a tea to clear lung congestion, ameliorate whooping cough, prevent nausea, and break fevers. The young pods were used for food.

The people of the Ojibwa nation, guided by their visions and trusting in their ancient traditions, had for thousands of years studied the plants that grew all around them. A remarkable Ojibwa medicine man gave a woman an herbal healing brew that cured her of breast cancer. The Grand Medicine Society of the Ojibwa had knowledge of herbal healing cures that was second to none throughout all of native America. The American herbal tradition owes a great deal to the Ojibwa and their sacred knowledge of the healing arts, which they had the kindness to pass on to settlers.

Long before science discovered the healing power of plants, or even believed that these powers existed, Native Americans were proficient healers, using the "green pharmacy" of Nature. For centuries, Native Americans had been treating a multitude of aches and pains with an herbal brew made from white willow bark. Today, we know a synthesized and refined product of willow bark as aspirin (acetylsalicylic acid).

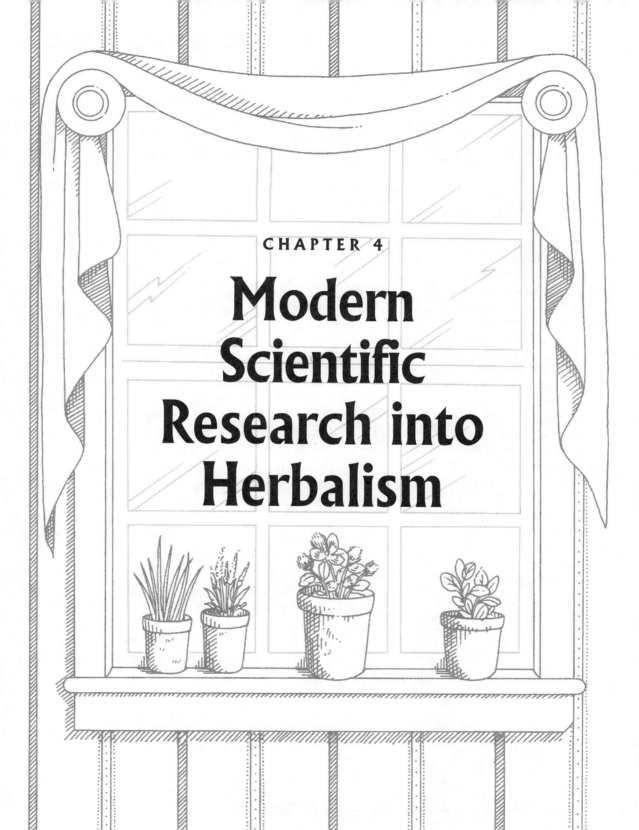

CHAPTER 4

Modern Scientific Research into Herbalism

AUTHOR'S NOTE

Clearly, it is impossible to cover the entire body of scientific evidence that has accumulated about herbs and their medicinal uses. This chapter is intended only to provide a brief overview, and to encourage the serious student of herbal medicine to go further in learning what scientific evidence is available—and there is much.

This book is not to be used for self-prescription: It is a guide to help the beginner through the thicket of often conflicting information about herbs and their uses as medicinal remedies. Any questions should be referred to proper authorities, such as those cited here, and anyone wishing to use herbs medicinally should do so in concert with a medical professional.

The crucial split between herbalism and orthodox medicine came with the unravelling of the effects of the foxglove, in 1785, by the English physician William Withering [who] had learned from herbalists that foxglove leaves could be a dramatic remedy for dropsy.... He discovered that the principal effect was in fact on the heart [which] eventually led to the discovery and purification of the active principles digitoxin and digoxin, now used in orthodox medicine as standard heart stimulants.

—The New Age Herbalist

Medical herbalism differs both from orthodox allopathic medicine and the typical home-based herbal remedies that people have used for centuries. For one thing, medical herbalism is based on the use of the entire plant. Another problem is that many herbs are prescribed for long-term and deep-seated problems and can take considerable time to have an effect. And yet another problem is that it is difficult to test and evaluate herbs used medically in the same fashion as orthodox pharmaceutical drugs are tested.

Today, several governments, most particularly that of Germany, are beginning to impose stricter conditions on the ingredients of commercially prepared herbal remedies and on how their usefulness is described and explained. However, despite the fact that there are difficulties presented in the testing of herbal remedies for medical purposes, there is a great need for herbal remedy research and analysis. Most of this need is being met by the German Commission E, of the *Bundesgesundheitsamt* (Federal Department of Health), which reviews the safety and efficacy of herbs and publishes the results of its findings in monographic form in the *Bundesanzeiger*, which is equivalent to the U.S. *Federal Register*. These German monographs constitute the most up-to-date and useful information available on the safety and efficacy of herbs and plants used medically, as drugs. They are often cited in various books and articles on herbalism.

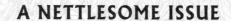

A NETTLESOME ISSUE

Scientists at the University of Frankfurt, the University of Dusseldorf, and St. Elizabeth's Clinic in Straubing, Germany, conducted studies of 40 people with sudden and severe attacks of arthritis pain. Half of those studied were given 200 milligrams of a nonsteroidal anti-inflammatory drug (NSAID) commonly used for arthritis pain, called Cataflam (diclofenac). The second half of those tested were given 50 milligrams of Cataflam along with 50 milligrams of stewed nettle leaves (cooking or drying nettle removes its stinging properties). The second group received only half the orthodox drug given to the first group.

Both groups experienced a lessening of pain and stiffness. However, the researchers were aware of a previous study in which people affected with arthritis were able to substitute half of their amounts of NSAIDs by adding 1,340 milligrams of dried, powdered nettle. At this writing, the researchers are attempting to discover if stinging nettle can help acute attacks of arthritis by itself, without being combined with NSAID drugs. They emphasize that anyone now taking medication should not make any changes, or add nettle, without consulting with their doctors.

AN AMERICAN ALLY

For anyone interested in delving further into the research of the German Commission E and its numerous monographs, Americans have the great good fortune to have a friend of this science in Mark Blumenthal, executive director of the American Botanical Council in Austin, Texas, Web site: *www.herbalgram.org*. Blumenthal has produced translations in English of the complete Commission E monographs, and now, for the first time, Americans can have ready access to the research, conclusions, and regulations endorsed by the German health authorities. This is extremely good news for those who are serious about herbal medicine and taking charge of their own health.

An example is the report on garlic in the May 1997 issue of the American magazine *Let's Live*. According to the report, garlic can cause a mild blood pressure lowering effect, particularly in hypertensive patients. The magazine article goes on to quote the *German Commission E Monograph* regarding garlic's action: ". . . lipid-lowering, inhibition of platelet aggregation, prolongation of bleeding and clotting time, enhancement of fibrinolytic activity." Noting that garlic must be taken for several months to receive optimum results, the article, following the German dosage recommendations, gives the following daily dosages for the different forms of garlic: powder (in capsule form)—400–1,200 mg; fresh—2–5 gm; oil—2–5 mg.

Valerian

According to Varro E. Tyler in his book *Honest Herbal*, the herb valerian is a good example of the different regulatory philosophies in Germany and the United States. The dried rhizome and roots of *Valerina officinalis L.* had been used as a tranquilizing agent for more than 1000 years, and valerian had enjoyed official status in the U.S. for 150 years, being included in *The United States Pharmacopoeia* from 1820 to 1942 and in *The National Formulary* from 1942 to 1950. Today, however, it is available in pharmacies only in the form of a tincture. "A pharmaceutical manufacturer would probably drop this product rather than spend the time and money necessary to prove its safety and efficacy—after ten centuries of use," says Tyler. Valerian today is sold as a "dietary supplement" in health food stores but has no official recognition.

In Germany, however, there are more than a hundred different proprietary drug products containing valerian or its active principles. Although German research has not yet been able to determine with certainty the exact composition of the components of valerian responsible for its calming and sedative properties, German health authorities have nonetheless declared the drug effective. They have pointed out that it is free from side effects, noting that when used as recommended, it has an advantage over synthetics, which mimic it.

Another calming herb, kava, has been studied by German researchers, who have demonstrated that the herb is a safe, non-addictive antianxiety medicine that is as effective as such drugs as Valium, which are prescribed for anxiety and tension.

In addition, the *British Journal of Phytotherapy* published a study showing kava extract has been shown to have the following pharmacological effects:

- Sedative and hypnotic
- Muscle-relaxing and anticonvulsant
- Antifungal
- Relaxing smooth muscle (e.g., that of the uterus)

The journal reported that although excessive use of kava can cause dizziness and grogginess, when used at the prescribed dosages, kava is safe: "The use of a standardized extract of kava equivalent to a daily dose of 210 mg of kava lactones did not result in adverse effects during up to eight weeks of continuous use."

Another much studied herb used to treat depression and related ills is St. John's wort (also known as hypericum). Researchers in Munich, Germany, conducted a methodical review of 23 randomized trials. They examined its effect on 1,757 people who suffered mild to moderately severe depressive symptoms. Their conclusion was that St. John's wort works as well for the treatment of mild to moderately severe depression as do standard pharmaceutical drugs prescribed as antidepressants. Says Donald J. Brown, N.D., a naturopathic physician in Seattle, Washington, and the author of *Herbal Prescriptions for Better Health*:

> *For women using St. John's wort for mild to moderate depression, it works as well as prescription antidepressants . . . [It] has none of the side effects that prescription antidepressants do. And it costs significantly less to use than Prozac—about 30 or 40 cents a day compared to about $4 a day for Prozac . . . When it comes to effectively treating mild to moderate depression with alternative therapies, St. John's wort is in a class by itself.*

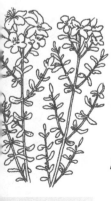

St. John's Wort

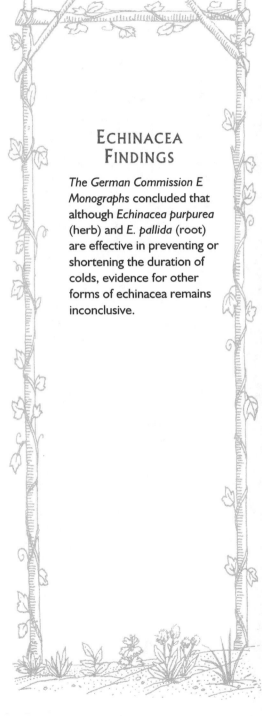

ECHINACEA FINDINGS

The German Commission E Monographs concluded that although *Echinacea purpurea* (herb) and *E. pallida* (root) are effective in preventing or shortening the duration of colds, evidence for other forms of echinacea remains inconclusive.

MEDIEVAL HERBAL WARFARE

The battle between the orthodox medical establishment and the herbal enthusiasts is nothing new. Renegade physicians such as William Turner wrote in English so that "the apothecaries and old wives that gather herbs" would know which plants physicians referred to in their Latin prescriptions, declaring he would not put "many a good man by ignorance in jeopardy of his life."

As medicine came more and more under the control of the "regular," or academic, physicians, the battles between them and the traditional "herb wives" raged throughout the 17th and 18th centuries. We all know who won.

Of interest to women is the German Commission E's approval of the herb black cohosh for premenstrual discomfort, difficult or painful menstruation, and menopausal ailments. In one clinical trial, 110 menopausal women were given either 8 milligrams of a dried black cohosh extract or a placebo. Researchers speculate that the herb has an estrogenic action and therefore reduces such symptoms as hot flashes, anxiety, and depression. The studies showed no side effects nor any link to increased risk of breast cancer, but the herb is contraindicated for use in pregnant or lactating women.

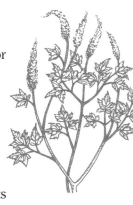

Black Cohosh

Many herbs are approved drugs in developed nations other than Germany—for example, Canada, Australia, and Britain—but FDA regulations make drug approval untenable for profit-motivated pharmaceutical companies who cannot patent herbal medicines in the United States. However, the Dietary Supplement Health and Education Act of 1994 (DSHEA) does permit herbal product supplements to be labeled with limited claims, which provide consumers with useful information about the proper use and the intended effects of these products.

Congress has, through DSHEA, actually set a tougher safety standard for supplements, including herbal remedies, than for pharmaceutical drugs, which can be sold even if they present significant risks through side effects.

Today, the climate is changing, and the demands of an ever-increasing group of enthusiastic herbal users who seek access to quality-guaranteed products, including accurate information about them, cannot be ignored forever by the regulatory bodies of the United States and its Congress.

In an interesting statement, published in the May/June 1999 issue of *Herbs for Health*, Rob McCaleb—founder and president of the Herb Research Foundation, a nonprofit educational organization in Boulder, Colorado—who lectures and publishes widely on the topic of medicinal herbs, says:

GREEN TEA

The research on green tea and green tea extract is extensive—and impressive. Here are some findings thus far:

- Countries that have a high consumption of green tea had lower rates of cancer than countries that do not consume much green tea.
- Green tea can block the development of angiogenesis—the new blood vessels needed by tumors in order for their cells to colonize and grow. Animal studies showed that the consumption of two or three cups of green tea daily was sufficient to significantly suppress tumor growth.
- Smokers who drink green tea—only about three cups daily—had less occurrence of lung damage than those who do not.
- Green tea extract can inhibit bacteria that cause periodontal disease and cavities; as a mouth rinse, it can reduce plaque.
- Women over the age of 40 who were not cigarette smokers and who drank five or more cups of green tea daily had half the incidence of stroke as those who drank less.
- Green tea contains catechins, which inhibit the proliferation of smooth muscle cells lining blood vessels, a process that can help prevent atherosclerosis and heart disease.
- The consumption of ten cups of green tea (or more) daily can protect against liver damage (from alcohol and other toxins).

HERBAL HELP ON-LINE

Access HerbDotCom's on-line herb library at *www.herb.com* to get advice from professionals and find out everything there is to know about all sorts of plants. Or you can "Ask Dr. Weil" at *chi.pathfinder.com/drweil/*. Andrew Weil, M.D., has archived according to date all of his findings, which guarantees the latest research information.

୨ ୬

ADDITIONAL READING

For a thorough—even exhaustive—explication of German medicine, its history, and its present-day status, see Chapter 9 of *Herbs Against Cancer* by Ralph W. Moss, Ph.D.

The Herb Research Foundation has more than 200,000 scientific articles and summaries in its files covering thousands of herbs. Among those papers are many that I think everyone simply assumes do not exist. For example, many herbs and their constituents have been researched using typical toxicological protocols, mutagenicity assays, multigeneration rodent studies, and so on. In many cases they also have been subjected to varying degrees of pharmacological analysis, which results from their use as medicines. This kind of research does not exist for foods. The most popular herbs now have clinical trials from Europe and Asia, and clinical cases in the thousands or millions under medical supervision. And, lest we forget, most botanicals have been widely used by dozens of generations of humans without apparent harm, which may be the best safety evidence available.

Furthermore, the DSHEA permits third-party literature, such as articles, book chapters, scientific reports, and so forth, to support the sale of herbal and dietary supplements without this being considered "drug labeling." However, the information given cannot be false or misleading, nor can it promote any specific product or commercial producer of any product.

NIH HERBAL DATA ON-LINE

If you want to see for yourself what the current state of scientific research is on herbs and other supplements, you can visit the new database *www.dietary-supplements.info.nih.gov* created by the Office of Dietary Supplements at the National Institutes of Health, which maintains a list of credible scientific studies on herbs, and everything else that is classified as "dietary supplements."

Called International Bibliographic Information on Dietary Supplements (IBIDS), the site permits you to search at no charge on hundreds of topics—just name your herb. With one mouse click, IBIDS will research your chosen herb in medical, botanical, and pharmaceutical databases, and display a list of relevant studies.

You can "save" study titles and summaries and send them to your e-mail account. The site also offers links to over a thousand medical and scientific journals that provide you with the entire text of any study you choose. And even better news comes from IBIDS coordinator Terri Krakower, Ph.D., who says that a set of peer-reviewed "fact sheets" that "interpret the scientific jargon in those reports" will soon be available on-line as well.

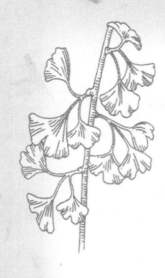

Part Two

THE HERBAL
PHARMACY

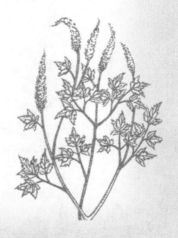

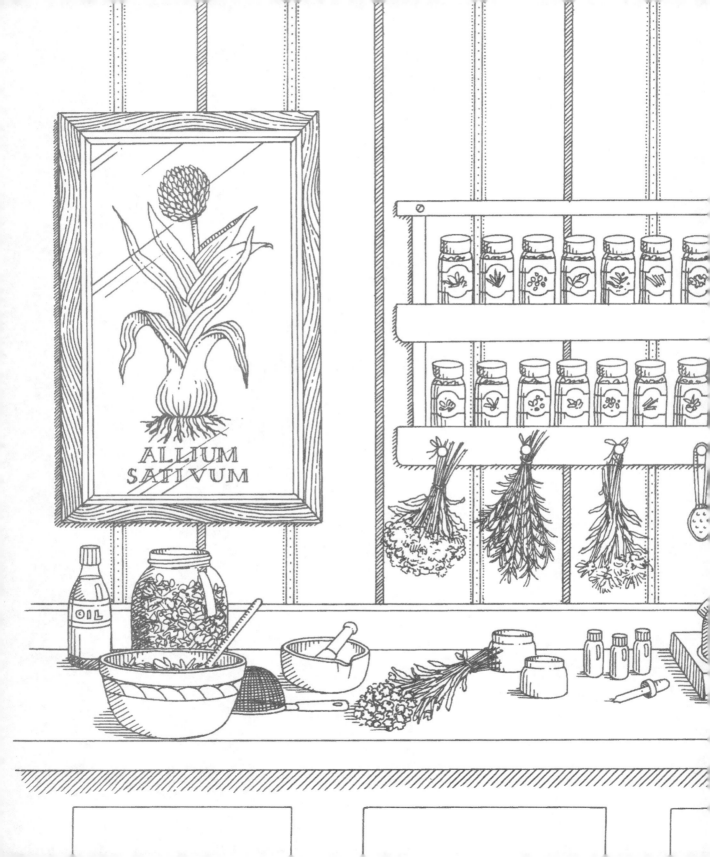

ALLIUM
SATIVUM

OIL

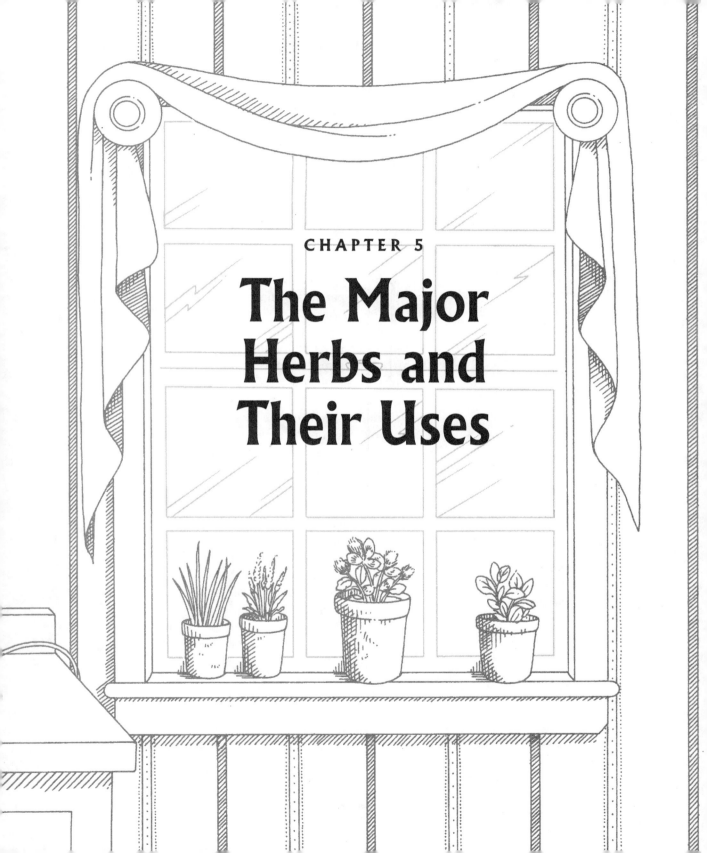

CHAPTER 5

The Major Herbs and Their Uses

DO YOUR HOMEWORK

- There is an abundance of information on herbs in bookstores and on the Internet.

- Talk to your physician about herbal therapy and don't ever self-prescribe without a professional diagnosis.

- Keep your doctor advised of all drugs and supplements, including herbals, that you take.

- Buy only from reputable manufacturers: The label should include the company's address, batch and lot numbers, expiration date, and recommended dosage.

- If you experience *any* side effects, discontinue use at once and consult your physician.

From food are born all creatures, which live upon food and after death return to food. Food is the chief of all things. It is therefore said to be the medicine of all diseases of the body.

—THE UPANISHAD, c. 500 B.C.

The current separation of plants into separate categories—herbs, vegetables, fruits, even weeds—is a recent occurrence in the history of how and what the world's peoples eat and have eaten. The 17th-century cook would have considered cabbage, carrots, and cucumbers to be "kitchen herbs," just as well as marigolds and parsley, thyme, marjoram, and other plants we today consider to be "herbs."

It is no longer common knowledge that the active constituents, such as alkaloids or saponins, of what we label today as "herbs" are also to be found in fruits and vegetables, which, therefore, also can have therapeutic qualities.

Thus, though herbs have played a vital role in the healing traditions of all cultures from the most ancient to modern, the alternative way of looking at health care, of which herbs form a large part, is as valid today as it was 5000 years ago.

There are literally thousands of plants known for medicinal properties, as well as many more—especially in our disappearing rain forests—that have not been investigated by Western scientific methods but are known to natives of these cultures. Of this great natural pharmacy, we will cover here the most common, most effective, and most readily available plants used as remedies. Some of these you will recognize as common to the kitchen, some to the garden, others as specific to particular ailments. Others will be new or unknown to you. Whatever your level of interest and knowledge of herbal use, this tour through Nature's great medicinal lore will be an adventure.

There's hardly anywhere on earth that doesn't have its share of plants known for their beneficial properties to human beings. Most of these are

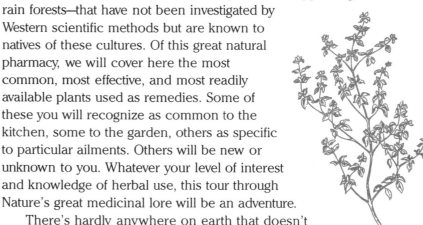

Thyme

quite humble, growing along roadsides or in fields, often mis-judged as "weeds." Others are cultivars with ancient histories.

An A to Z of Common Medicinal Herbs

The following entries each contain descriptions of the herb, or plant, and list both the common and botanical names. Medicinal uses are noted. It is important to realize that herbs generally affect the entire bodily system in a holistic manner while at the same time are being used for specific body parts or ailments.

Instructions for usual dosage for the average adult are included as are the most suitable methods of application (i.e., oral or topical). Though most people today buy their herbs already prepared either in capsule or tablet form, or as ointments, salves, or lotions, for those interested in making their own preparations, instructions for doing so are included.

The selection of herbs here are generally Western, deriving from ancient, European, and Native American traditions. Some Asian herbs are now common to the West—such as ginger, cinnamon, and ginseng. (Specifically Chinese herbs as well as those from other cultures around the world are considered in Chapter 6.)

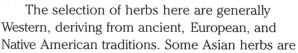

Coriander

Of the herbs listed here, most are considered reasonably safe when recommendations for usage are followed. As with any substance, excess can do harm, but there is little harm to be found with herbs when they are administered properly. When buying packaged herbal products, choose a reliable brand and follow the manufacturer's directions concerning dosage. Such directions may vary from manufacturer to manufacturer due to factors such as potency, so always be sure to follow the label directions.

If you are preparing your own concentrate of herbs, follow the recommendations given here or, again, on the label of the product you purchase. Some people like to buy herbs in bulk and make their own teas or infusions (see Chapter 11).

HERBS: A DEFINITION

The *Concise Oxford Dictionary* defines an herb as (a) any nonwoody seed-bearing plant that dies down to the ground after flowering or (b) any plant with leaves, seeds, or flowers used for flavoring, food, medicine, scent, and so on. And all of us understand the simple commonsensical definition of herbs to be basically anything that grows and is useful.

IT STICKS WITH YOU

An herb popular during the 14th century in Europe to treat leprosy was called "burdock" (because of its hooked burrs that stuck to clothing). Traditionally used as a blood purifier, it was made into folk brews, or wine, and used for indigestion. The Chinese use the seeds, called *niu bang zi,* to dispel "wind and heat evils."

Burdock has a long and worldwide history as a cancer treatment. St. Hildegard mixed up a potion with it as an ingredient to use against the disease. Current studies suggest that the nun was not off the mark. An article in *Chemotherapy* quoted research that identified the chemical arctigenin as an "inhibitor of experimental tumor growth."

When using herbs to treat any specific ailment for which you are also consulting a medical doctor, be sure to advise him or her that you are using herbs in addition to any medicines prescribed for your condition. Today, many doctors are becoming aware of the benefits of herbal use and are often open to a combination of treatments. For example, a person being treated for arthritis is advised to take ginger, an ancient remedy with a safety record thousands of years old. Few medical doctors would object to such a patient ingesting ginger—but it's important to keep your medical practitioner "in the loop" if you begin taking herbs for specific conditions for which you are already being treated.

Some herbs are reputed to have anticancer properties; these are especially popular in Europe and other countries. However, anyone who is under the care of an oncologist should never discontinue conventional treatment nor use any herbs in conjunction with it without the approval of his or her medical advisor.

Although many herbs can safely be given to children, the wise course for parents is to first check with a qualified pediatrician before administering herbal remedies to a child.

In addition, pregnant women should not take herbal preparations without consulting with their obstetricians.

These caveats being given, let me emphasize the long history of safe use of herbs in the treatment of a myriad of human ailments. Many herbs are familiar to us as ingredients we use in cooking—and in fact all of the herbs and spices used today for flavoring were originally prized for their healing properties and ability to preserve food.

As we are complex beings, functioning on physical, mental, emotional, and spiritual planes, our health is likewise a complex issue. Being holistic, we respond to what is also holistic, which is why herbs are beneficial to our entire systems. The Western medical tradition treats us as mere body parts—your liver may malfunction and the doctor treats it as if it were unconnected to the rest of your body/mind/spirit. Herbalists, on the other hand, as do homeopaths and other alternative healers, look at the whole person. In some traditions, for example, the liver is considered the seat of the emotions. It's important to bear this in mind as you study and use herbs.

ALFALFA (*medicago sativa*)

Common names: Buffalo herb, lucerne, purple medic
Medicinal part: Leaves

Description: A perennial plant, alfalfa is widely cultivated and can be found wild in fields and low valleys. An erect, smooth stem grows to a height of 12 to 18 inches, producing trifoliate leaves and blue or purple flowers that grow in racemes from June to August. The seeds are in spirally coiled pods.

Most often considered merely as fodder for cattle, this useful plant with an ancient history as a healing herb fell from public favor after the Civil War only to return to our attention in the 1970s in the form of its sprouts, as a popular salad ingredient. However, alfalfa has a long history as an adjunct to human health. Originally discovered by the Arabs, who called alfalfa "the father of all foods," its leaves—which contain its real healing properties—are rich in minerals and other nutrients, including calcium, magnesium, potassium, and beta carotene (recently touted by Dr. Andrew Weil as a powerful antioxidant against "free radicals" that roam the body as toxins). There are indications that alfalfa may reduce "bad" cholesterol, thus helping to prevent heart disease and some types of strokes.

Noticing that their cattle consumed alfalfa eagerly, ancient Chinese farmers began cooking the herb's tender young leaves as a vegetable and discovered that it was an effective appetite stimulant and also that it was useful for digestive disorders. Alfalfa has been used to treat ulcers.

The Spanish conquistadors introduced alfalfa to the New World as a forage crop for their horses, especially in the Great Plains area, where the American pioneers took it up as a crop. Our pioneering ancestors used alfalfa to treat a multitude of ailments including arthritis, boils, scurvy (a condition brought on by a lack of vitamin C), and urinary and bowel difficulties. Our foremothers used alfalfa to bring on menstruation.

Today, in applications never before considered, alfalfa has come to the attention of modern-day scientists who have discovered that it can be an agent in the treatment of heart disease, stroke, and cancer—the top three causes of death in the United States. However, despite its reputation as a treatment for ulcers, no

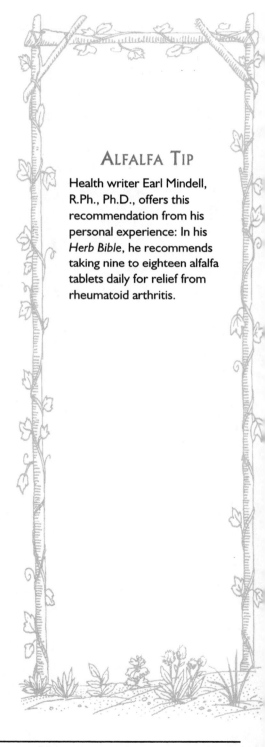

ALFALFA TIP

Health writer Earl Mindell, R.Ph., Ph.D., offers this recommendation from his personal experience: In his *Herb Bible*, he recommends taking nine to eighteen alfalfa tablets daily for relief from rheumatoid arthritis.

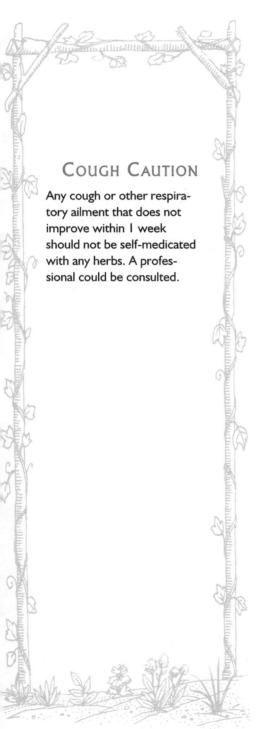

COUGH CAUTION

Any cough or other respiratory ailment that does not improve within 1 week should not be self-medicated with any herbs. A professional could be consulted.

scientific evidence supports this traditional use. The use of alfalfa leaves has not been proven to promote menstruation, but it may well have been the seeds (which contain two chemicals, stachydrine and homostachydrine that can bring on menstruation and/or cause miscarriage) that pioneer women used, possibly to end an unwanted pregnancy. Alfalfa seeds are to be avoided entirely, especially by anyone with an autoimmune problem.

Alfalfa leaf is on the FDA's list of herbs generally regarded as safe, but it should be used in medicinal amounts only with your doctor's approval. If the condition for which you are using the herb does not improve significantly within two weeks, or if you experience any side effects—such as upset stomach or diarrhea—stop use.

Dosage

Capsules or tablets: Take three to six daily, or follow the manufacturer's instructions on the label.

Bulk dried leaves: Steep 1 tablespoon in 8 ounces of hot water for 5 to 15 minutes. Drink 1 to 3 cups of the tea daily.

ALLSPICE (*Pimenta officinalis, P. diocia*)

Common names: Clove pepper, Jamaica pepper, pimento

Medicinal part: Fruit: the mature but still green berry.

Description: Allspice, the dried berry of the pimento, comes from an evergreen tree that grows as high as 40 feet. Native to the West Indies and Central America, it is now cultivated in South America and Mexico. Its large, leathery, oblong leaves with prominent veins on the underside are followed by small white flowers that produce clusters of half-inch berries from June to August. When ripe, the fruit is a sweet berry, but when used for allspice, it is picked while unripe and then dried. Primarily a Caribbean tree, it is not grown in the United States.

Many of us, if we know allspice at all, know it only as a spicy ingredient in Caribbean food. If we have visited the islands, we've heard it called pimento, its local name, which we think of a large red bell pepper often used to flavor cheese spreads. But the Caribbean pimento, which we call allspice, is far more interesting than as a mere flavoring for exotic food.

THE MISTAKE COLUMBUS MADE

It is one of the ironies of history that at a time of avid exploration for spices and gold, Christopher Columbus sailed right past one of the richest spice treasures in the New World—not once, but twice! As he roamed the Caribbean Islands, he saw "trees of a thousand kinds, all laden with fruit which the Admiral believed to be spiceries and nutmeg —but they were not ripe and he did not recognize them." Unfortunately for Columbus, he was ignorant of botany, or he would have recognized the allspice trees, which bear one of the most valued of all true spices.

Later Spanish explorers encountered the trees when they were covered with ripe berries. As dried allspice berries look identical to large peppercorns, the Spaniards took them to be pepper, naming the spice "pimento," which the botanists translated to *Pimenta officinalis*, still its scientific name. In Jamaica, where allspice grows most lavishly and is an ingredient of almost everything, it is still known as pimento, and that is how the U.S. Customs Department lists it in its records.

Seemingly mundane today, allspice has a romantic past, playing an important part in the era of melodramatic cloak-and-dagger derring-do of the 17th-century pirate days. As such swashbuckling robber sailors as Henry Morgan and Calico Jack Rackham plundered ships along the Spanish Main, allspice preserved the meats with which they stocked their galleys while at sea. The meat, cured by smoking and seasoning with allspice, was called boucan, and it was their dependence on this food source that gave them the name boucaneers, from which we get buccaneers.

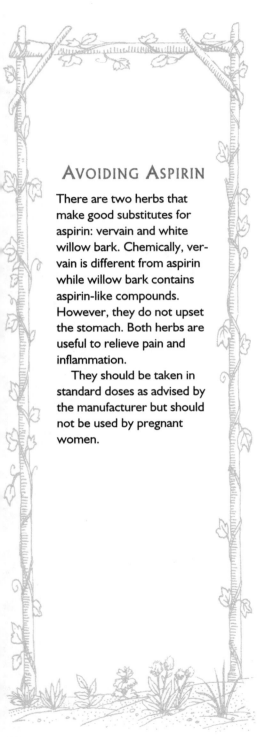

AVOIDING ASPIRIN

There are two herbs that make good substitutes for aspirin: vervain and white willow bark. Chemically, vervain is different from aspirin while willow bark contains aspirin-like compounds. However, they do not upset the stomach. Both herbs are useful to relieve pain and inflammation.

They should be taken in standard doses as advised by the manufacturer but should not be used by pregnant women.

Combining the flavors of cinnamon, pepper, juniper, and clove—hence the rubric allspice—it is used as a digestive aid, pain reliever, and anesthetic. Different islanders use it for different purposes: Jamaicans make a hot tea from allspice for colds, stomach upsets, and menstrual cramps; in Costa Rica, it is used for indigestion, flatulence, and as a treatment for diabetes; Guatemalans crush allspice berries for an external application to heal bruises and joint and muscle pain; in Cuba it is considered a tonic.

Allspice's secret ingredient is an oil that is the source of all of its healing properties. Allspice oil is rich in the chemical eugenol, which is also found in cloves and other healing herbs. It is thought that eugenol promotes the activity of digestive enzymes. Studies have proved that eugenol is an effective topical pain reliever, bearing witness to the Guatemalan tradition of treating painful joints and muscles with the crushed berries.

In this country and elsewhere, dentists use eugenol as a local anesthetic. It is an ingredient in a substance used on patients with sensitive or inflamed gums prior to cleaning the teeth, a process which can irritate the gums. Eugenol is also an ingredient in such over-the-counter products as Numizident and Benzodent, which are sold as toothache remedies. The pure oil of allspice may be used as a first-aid remedy by applying it directly to aching teeth or painful gums until professional help can be obtained. However, *never* ingest the oil directly; a small amount can cause nausea, vomiting, and even convulsions.

Allspice is generally sold in whole-berry and powdered form for cooking purposes and so is readily available in the supermarket or from a herb and spice supplier (see Resources).

Considered a mild antioxidant, allspice may help prevent the cell damage that scientists claim leads to cancer. However, scientific tests suggest that eugenol may be a weak factor in growth of tumors. Since this dual factor exists (as it does with many healing herbs), persons with any cancer history should not use allspice medicinally.

Allspice is on the FDA's list of herbs generally regarded as safe. Thus, healthy adults, except for pregnant and nursing women, can safely use allspice in the recommended amounts.

As with all herbs, if the condition does not improve in two weeks, or if you experience unpleasant side effects, discontinue use and consult your doctor.

Dosage

Oil of allspice: For toothache or gum pain, apply the oil directly, using a cotton swab, 1 drop only. Do not swallow the oil.

Powder for tea: As a digestive aid, use 1 or 2 teaspoons of allspice powder per cup of boiling water. Allow to steep for 10 to 20 minutes; then strain. You can drink up to 3 cups per day.

ALOE VERA (*aloe barbadensis* Mill; family Liliaceae)

Common names: Cape, Barbados, Curaiao, Socotrine, and Zanzibar Aloe

Medicinal parts: Gel from inside the thick succulent leaves and the juice (latex) extracted from specialized cells of the leaves' inner skins

Description: A member of the lily family, aloe vera has over three hundred species of which *A. barbadensis* is the most familiar to us. Its cactus-like, long, narrow, gray-green, prickly edge leaves yield a sticky gel when cut open. A perennial, the plant grows best in sandy soils in dry, sunny climates. Today it can be found throughout the American Southwest, in California, in Mexico, and in Central and South America. Except for places with extremely cold climates, some species of aloe grows almost everywhere.

The Romans were not the only ones who considered aloe vera to be a healing plant. In order to guarantee a supply for treating his soldier's wounds, Alexander the Great conquered the island Socotra, where aloe was first cultivated. From as far back as ancient Egypt, there is evidence of aloe's healing powers. The *Papyrus Ebers*, discovered in 1873 by German Egyptologist, Georg Ebers, contains recipes for preparing aloe. Queen Cleopatra, known for her beauty, used aloe as a skin moisturizer, no doubt a great boon in the hot, dry climate of Egypt.

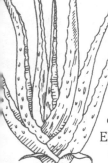
Aloe Vera

PLINY THE ELDER ON ALOE

"There are many uses for [aloe], but the chief is to relax the bowels, for it is almost the only laxative that is also a stomach tonic."

GROW YOUR OWN ALOE

It's easy to grow your own aloe vera plant indoors. It requires sun but will tolerate filtered light or shade; it will also tolerate poor soil. Being a succulent, it needs little water. A hardy plant, it will nonetheless suffer from poor drainage and temperatures below 40 degrees.

N IS
FOR DOCTOR

Naturopaths, doctors who are fully licensed as N.D.s, generally recommend natural approaches for the treatment of health problems.

To find a naturopath in your area, contact the

American Association of Naturopathic Physicians
601 Valley Street, Suite 105, Seattle, Washington 98109

or you can telephone them at

206-298-0125 or visit their Web site *www.naturopathic.org.*

The association will send you a national directory of their members for the nominal charge of $5.

Aloe's use as a purgative was also prevalent as the early Egyptians believed disease came from food and that the body, therefore, needed regular purges, an idea that came down through the Middle Ages, when it was a favored laxative, to the present day. Many herbalists still prepare "cleansing" combinations, and regular abstinence from food for short periods of time is still popular.

The Greek physician Dioscorides recommended aloe externally for wounds, hemorrhoids, and ulcers, and believed that it could stop hair loss; Pliny recommended it both as an external healer for wounds, bruises, and irritations and as an internal cleanser, tonic, and jaundice remedy.

Contemporary herbalists recommend aloe primarily for external use—for wounds, burns, scalds, scrapes, and sunburn. Scientific evidence of aloe's healing properties was reported in an American medical journal in 1935. A woman who suffered from X-ray burns was successfully treated with aloe gel squeezed directly from leaves cut from the plant. Since then, other studies have supported aloe's wonderful healing ability, especially for first- and second-degree burns, as well as minor skin irritations such as poison ivy rash. Apparently it also combats infection from skin injuries; studies have shown it to be effective against many bacteria that can cause infection of a wound.

Psoriasis, a chronic skin disease that forms scaly red itchy patches and has long resisted treatment, was shown, in a study conducted at the Malmo University Hospital in Sweden, to improve by topically applying aloe vera extract (0.5 percent) in a water-based cream. And, in 1995, the FDA approved an aloe vera-based gel disk, researched at Baylor College of Dentistry, containing acemannan hydrogel, that reduces irritation from mouth sores and heals them faster that conventional methods.

However, aloe vera should be used with extreme caution as a laxative. It contains aloin (from the outer rind of the leaf), which is classified as a drug by the FDA. Aloe latex should *never* be taken by pregnant or lactating women. In general, only the gel from the inner leaf, usually in liquid form, should be ingested.

Aloe gel is safe for external use unless there is an allergic reaction. As with all herbal remedies, it is best used in consultation with your doctor. If a skin wound fails to heal promptly, seek medical advice.

Dosage

Gel: 1 to 2 ounces per application, up to 1 pint daily. Or break off a leaf from your own plant and smear the gel on the burn or wound several times a day.

Liquid: Aloe vera in liquid form is available in health food stores. It is considered helpful for some ulcerative and gastrointestinal problems. Begin with a small amount, up to $1/4$ cup. Monitor your body's reaction carefully. If it helps and you tolerate it well, you can gradually increase the amount ingested daily.

ANGELICA (*Angelica archangelica*)

Common names: Wild celery, masterwort; in China *dang-gui*
Medicinal parts: Roots, leaves, seeds
Description: Resembling the common vegetable celery, angelica grows to a height of 8 feet—hence its common name wild celery. A biennial, it dies after producing its seeds and is reproduced from seeds or root divisions.

Angelica is a source of controversy between herbalists and scientists, who dismiss it as medically worthless. Some go so far as to warn that it can be toxic due to the component *psoralens*, which, on contact with the skin, may cause photosensivitity to the sun, resulting in skin damage. However, angelica root has been approved in Germany where it is used for loss of appetite, flatulence, and mild gastrointestinal tract spasms.

Angelica has a long history of several thousand years of use, both for medical and magical purposes. For over a thousand years, European peasants used necklaces made of angelica leaf to protect their children's health as well as to ward off evil. Supposed to cause witches to flee, its presence in a woman's cupboard or garden was used as proof of innocence against charges of practicing witchcraft.

THE HERB OF ANGELS

As angelica often blooms around May 8, the feast day of St. Michael the Archangel—which gives the herb its Latin name of *archangelica*—it is known as the "Herb of Angels."

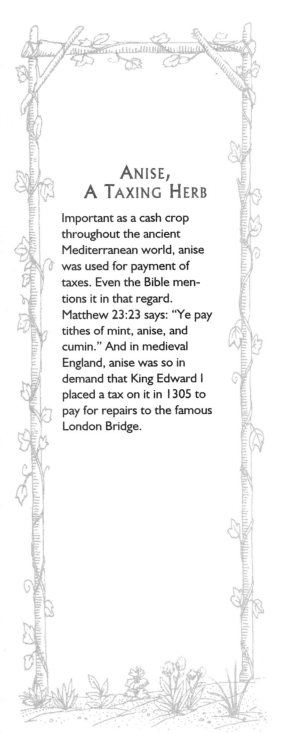

ANISE, A TAXING HERB

Important as a cash crop throughout the ancient Mediterranean world, anise was used for payment of taxes. Even the Bible mentions it in that regard. Matthew 23:23 says: "Ye pay tithes of mint, anise, and cumin." And in medieval England, anise was so in demand that King Edward I placed a tax on it in 1305 to pay for repairs to the famous London Bridge.

Contemporary herbalists usually suggest angelica for digestive problems or excess production of mucus. Indeed, German researchers have discovered that angelica relaxes the windpipe, which suggests it is of value in treating respiratory ailments such as colds, flu, bronchitis, and asthma. German researchers have also found that angelica relaxes the intestines, which may be the reason it is effective as a digestive aid. In Asia, it is traditionally used as an arthritis remedy, and Japanese researchers report that angelica has anti-inflammatory properties. Chinese investigators in preliminary research reports suggest that angelica increases the red blood cell count and the blood's clotting ability, but the full results are not yet in. Even though one day angelica may be a treatment for clotting impairment, it should be avoided by anyone at risk for heart disease. The Chinese research also suggests angelica may improve liver function in cases of cirrhosis and chronic hepatitis, but this research is preliminary, and at present angelica cannot be recommended for liver problems.

Angelica's antispasmodic action relieves menstrual cramps. It also has a warming effect on the body, promoting circulation to the extremities, a useful remedy for those suffering from cold hands and feet.

The FDA includes angelica in its list of herbs generally regarded as safe for healthy adults (except pregnant or lactating women), when used as recommended, so long as they have no history of cancer, heart attack, or photosensitivity.

Dosage

Infusion: Use 1 teaspoon of powdered seeds or leaves per cup of boiling water; steep 10 to 20 minutes.

Decoction: Use 1 teaspoon of powdered roots per cup of water. Simmer 2 minutes, then let stand for 15 minutes. Drink up to 2 cups daily. The bitter taste may be sweetened with honey.

Commercial extracts: Follow the package directions.

Caution: Do not give full strength to children under 2 or to adults over 65. Dilute and decrease strength if appropriate.

ANISE (*Pimpinella anisum*)

Common names: Aniseed, sweet cumin

Medicinal part: Fruit (called seeds)

Description: An annual, anise can reach 2 feet in height. A member of the parsley family, its smooth stem supports fern-like leaves in many leaflets. Clusters of tiny white or yellow flowers bloom in midsummer and produce the little ribbed fruits in late summer.

Although most of us know anise best as a flavoring agent, the aromatic fruit, so small it looks like seeds, has a long history with many uses, both cosmetic (for perfume) and medicinal. The ancient Greeks used it to prevent seizures, and Hippocrates, known as the "father of medicine," advised its use to clear mucus from the respiratory passages. In colonial times, anise was so valued that each settler in Virginia was required by law to plant six anise seeds.

Anise is particularly used as a digestive aid, and in Roman times it was a component of a dual-purpose cake called *mustaceum* which was both a dessert and a digestive aid, a must after the huge Roman banquets. Early English herbalist, John Gerard, recommended it for hiccups. It is also a traditional herb used by nursing mothers to increase milk flow, and recent studies have revealed that anise contains chemicals similar to the female hormone estrogen, which may account for this use. As anise has only mild estrogenic activity, it can be used to relieve menopausal discomforts.

Today as always, herbalists recommend anise as an expectorant for cough and bronchitis. Modern studies have shown the herb to contain chemicals that serve to loosen bronchial secretions. Studies have also supported its use as a digestive aid against upset stomach and flatulence by confirming the presence of another chemical, anethole, which promotes digestion.

Dosage

Infusion: Use 1 teaspoon of crushed anise seeds per cup of boiling water; steep for 10 to 20 minutes and strain. Drink up to 3 cups daily.

Tincture: Use ½ to 1 teaspoon up to 3 times daily, or follow label directions on commercial products.

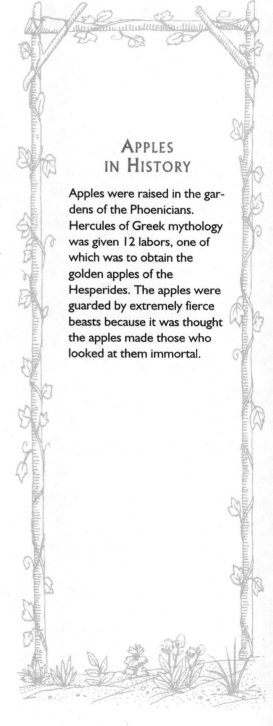

APPLES IN HISTORY

Apples were raised in the gardens of the Phoenicians. Hercules of Greek mythology was given 12 labors, one of which was to obtain the golden apples of the Hesperides. The apples were guarded by extremely fierce beasts because it was thought the apples made those who looked at them immortal.

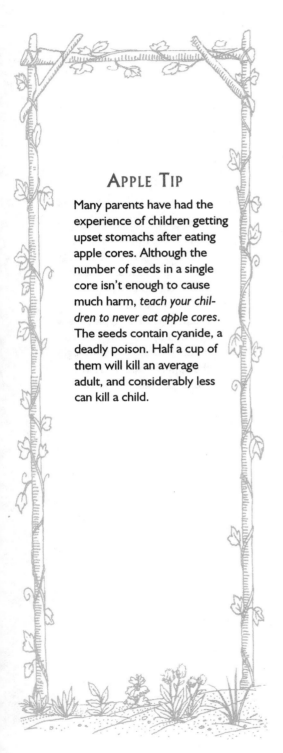

APPLE

Common names: None

Medicinal parts: Fruit pulp and skin; *never* eat seeds

Description: Who can describe an apple? In shape, it can be round like a McIntosh or oblong like the Delicious. In size, it can vary from a 2-inch crabapple to a 6-inch Rome Beauty. The flesh may be white as a Wealthy, yellow as a Golden Delicious, crisp as a Northern Spy, mellow as a Baldwin, sweet as a Grimes Golden, or tart as a new Winesap. The apple's skin is thin and glossy, ranging in color from bright or russet red to yellow or bright green.

Apple

It might seem odd to include the apple in a book about herbal remedies, but originally, all plant-based remedies were considered to be "herbal," and the apple not only has a venerable tradition as a healing agent but also has recently been scientifically approved as such. We've all heard the old adage that "an apple a day keeps the doctor away," and recent studies support this nostrum—especially if the doctor in question is a gastroenterologist, cardiologist, or oncologist. Studies have shown that apples are good for treating both diarrhea and constipation and may be instrumental as a preventative for heart disease, some types of stroke, and even cancer.

The active ingredient in apple pulp is pectin, a soluble form of fiber. As an agent against diarrhea, pectin acts with the intestinal bacteria to create a soothing, protective coating for the irritated intestinal lining. One study shows pectin to be effective against diarrhea-causing bacteria, which explains why the "pectate" in the popular over-the-counter preparation for diarrhea. Kaopectate is pectin. For constipation, apple pectin adds bulk to the digestive system, which stimulates normal bowel contractions, making stool evacuation easier.

Pectin may be effective against heart disease and stroke because it helps reduce "bad" cholesterol by keeping it in the intestinal tract until it is eliminated. Fresh apples are especially recommended as a dessert in such cases. Also, according to the American Cancer Society, a high-fiber diet helps to prevent several forms of cancer, especially colon cancer. A study published in the *Journal of the National Cancer Institute* shows that pectin binds certain cancer-causing compounds in the colon, accelerating their removal from the body.

High-fiber diets are also recommended by physicians for their diabetic patients and several studies have shown that apple pectin can help control blood sugar levels in diabetics.

Apples are also used for internal cleansing. European studies indicate that apple pectin can help to eliminate lead, mercury, and other toxic heavy metals from the human body—so "an apple a day" is especially good advice for those living in polluted areas such as big inner cities. Eating raw apples also helps cleanse the teeth, an important health consideration, as many serious diseases have now been linked to unhealthy gums and teeth.

Not only does the tree's delicious fruit provide numerous health benefits, it gives us its leaves for use as a first-aid treatment for cuts and wounds. The leaves contain the antibiotic phloretin and can be crushed and pressed onto a cut or skin abrasion as a temporary measure.

Dosage

Use the entire fruit, peel and all, but *never* eat the seeds, which are poisonous. Unless you can obtain your apples from a certified organic source, wash them thoroughly in soap and water to remove pesticide residues; commercially produced apples are always raised with pesticides. Once cleaned, you can eat as many as you like, raw or cooked in various ways. Applesauce is a good treatment for diarrhea; a person suffering stomach upset may not want to eat raw food, and warm applesauce is soothing both to the tummy and the psyche.

ARNICA (*Arnica montana; Arnica fulgens* Pursh)
Common names: Arnica flowers, arnica rot, common arnica, leopardsbane, mountain arnica, mountain tobacco, wolfsbane
Medicinal parts: Flowers, rootstock
Description: A perennial, arnica is commonly found in the mountainous regions of Canada, the northern United States, and

LET THE HERB'S NAME FIT THE DISEASE

In colonial times, during the outbreak of a particularly nasty flu, which the settlers named "break bone fever" because the pain that accompanied it was so intense it felt like breaking bones, Native Americans introduced the settlers to a New World herbal cure. Thus, it was named "boneset" and became one of the most common home remedies of the 1800s. The entire plant was used to make a tea to combat colds and flu and it is still used for that purpose. Also, it provides a mild tonic effect in the elderly and can be useful as a mild laxative.

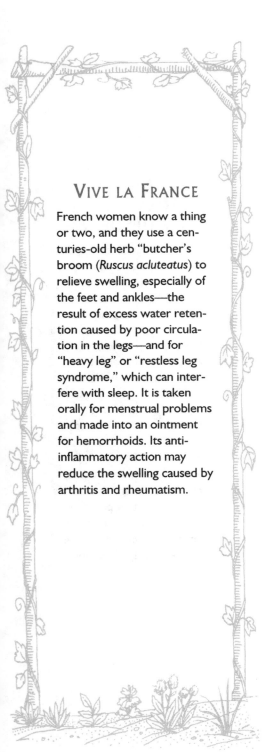

VIVE LA FRANCE

French women know a thing or two, and they use a centuries-old herb "butcher's broom (*Ruscus acluteatus*) to relieve swelling, especially of the feet and ankles—the result of excess water retention caused by poor circulation in the legs—and for "heavy leg" or "restless leg syndrome," which can interfere with sleep. It is taken orally for menstrual problems and made into an ointment for hemorrhoids. Its anti-inflammatory action may reduce the swelling caused by arthritis and rheumatism.

Europe. A horizontal, dark brown, branched rootstock produces a stem reaching to a height of 1 to 2 feet. The large, yellow, daisylike flowers appear from June to August.

Arnica's history as a medicinal plant is long. We know that Native Americans knew its healing properties at an early date, but not exactly when. In Europe, arnica's virtues were discovered before the end of the 16th century. The entire plant, including roots, was used for internal concoctions at that time, but today's modern herbalists are extremely cautious about its internal use, as an overdose can be fatal. External use is quite safe, however, and arnica is wonderful for healing wounds, bruises, and skin abrasions and irritations such as rashes. Commercial preparations of liniments are used for arthritis and sore muscles.

Arnica has been widely used for centuries as a home remedy for aches and bruises, but how or why it worked remained a mystery until 1981, when German researchers found that certain sesquiterpenoid lactones were the active agents. These were discovered to possess pharmacological properties that explained arnica's anti-inflammatory and analgesic effects, as well as some antibiotic action.

Note: One of these elements, helenalin, is known to be an allergen that causes contact dermatitis in some people. Therefore, if any negative reaction is noticed, the application of arnica should be discontinued at once.

Despite this drawback, arnica is approved in Germany for external use to treat hematomas, sprains, bruises, contusions, rheumatic pains of muscles and joints, and for edema caused by sprains and fractures. In the United States, commercially marketed arnica preparations are the best choice.

Dosage

Carefully follow manufacturer's directions on any over-the-counter preparations containing arnica. Do not attempt to prepare ointments or salves at home, as anything too strong will cause irritation. Do not apply arnica to skin that is broken, *and never take arnica internally unless you are under the supervision of a medical or homeopathic physician.*

ASPARAGUS (*Asparagus officinalis*)

Common name: Sparrow grass

Medicinal parts: Young shoots, seeds

Description: Most people are familiar with asparagus as a vegetable. It is a perennial plant, generally cultivated, but can also be found in the wild. The shoots are picked young in spring. A red berry fruit contains black seeds that ripen in August.

Though most of us consider asparagus only as a vegetable that signals the onset of spring, worldwide it has been highly regarded as a healing herb. In India, it is used to promote fertility, reduce menstrual cramping, and increase milk production in nursing mothers.

Primarily, however, asparagus is a potent diuretic. At the same time, it is highly nutritious, as it contains folic acid, which helps prevent anemia and which most Americans rarely get in sufficient quantity unless they take it as a supplement. It increases cellular activity in the kidneys, increasing the rate of urine production, and may also help with constipation because it contains indigestible fiber. Due to the anti-inflammatory action of the component steroidal glycocides, herbal healers recommend asparagus for rheumatism, especially the gouty type.

The seed in powdered form will calm an upset stomach. It is available from health food stores and by mail order.

Dosage

Fresh, raw, or cooked: Eat the young shoots; avoid buying those appearing brown or limp. They should be bright green and crisp enough to snap off the hard bottom end.

Seeds: Available in powdered form at health food stores. Take 1 teaspoon of powder dissolved in any liquid once a day.

ASTRAGALUS (*Astragalus membranaceous*)

Common names: Milk-vetch root, huang qi

Medicinal part: Root

Description: The astragalus root is a rhizome.

As astragalus's primary medical use is to strengthen the immune system, it is an important herb in today's world. Long

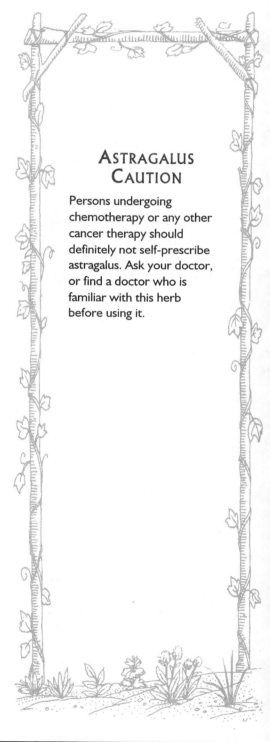

ASTRAGALUS CAUTION

Persons undergoing chemotherapy or any other cancer therapy should definitely not self-prescribe astragalus. Ask your doctor, or find a doctor who is familiar with this herb before using it.

used in Chinese herbal medicine, the August *Journal of the American Cancer Society* reported that astralagus strengthened the immune function of a large proportion of the patients studied. Dr. G. Mavligit at the University of Texas in Houston reported that an extract from astragalus helped restore normal immune function in cancer patients with impaired immunity. It is often given to those undergoing chemotherapy and radiation therapy, and research is ongoing to discover the full range of its medical properties.

As an immune system enhancer, it is recommended for colds as well as general resistance to disease. Also, it may help to reduce blood pressure by ridding the body of excess fluids.

Dosage
Capsules: Take 1 to 3 400-milligram capsules daily, or follow the manufacturer's directions on the label.

BALM (*Melissa officinalis*)
Common names: Lemon balm, bee balm, sweet balm, mellisa

Medicinal part: Leaves

Description: A perennial plant, balm is common in the Near East and the Mediterranean, but it has been naturalized in the United States. Cultivated as a culinary herb, it can be found wild in fields and gardens and along roadsides. Growing as high as 3 feet, its upright, hairy stem is branched. Balm flowers in clusters from pale yellow to rose color or blue-white in July and August. When bruised, the whole plant smells like lemon.

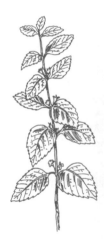

Lemon Balm

Called "bee balm" because bees love its fragrant flowers, and mellisa, Greek for "bee," balm has been a popular healing herb for 2000 years. The ancient Greek physician Dioscorides used it to apply to skin wounds, the Roman Pliny recommended it to stop bleeding, and 10th-century Arab doctors prescribed it for nervousness and anxiety.

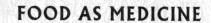

FOOD AS MEDICINE

Oats, olives, and onions may not technically belong to the category of herbs, but their beneficial properties should not be overlooked.

Oats are a marvelous source of energy, and oat bran is an excellent fiber that can reduce serum cholesterol. An oat extract can be used to relieve indigestion (10 to 20 drops up to three times daily). Used in the bath, oats are soothing to the skin and calming to the psyche.

Olives, long an essential part of the Mediterranean diet, are delicious, and their oil, high in monounsaturated fats, has recently hit the headlines because of its ability to reduce "bad" cholesterol in the blood. Dr. Andrew Weil recommends the exclusive use of olive oil for fat in the diet. Studies have shown that people who consume olive oil in preference to other fats have a lower incidence of heart disease. A small ball of cotton soaked in warmed olive oil and placed in the ear can relieve an earache.

Onions, traditionally known as "pot herbs," are a good source of allium, a substance also found in garlic. A study by the National Cancer Institute showed that those with diets high in allium vegetables are less prone to stomach cancer than those who avoid these vegetables.

Raw onion helps clear the sinus and nasal passages; salted onions are used to dry up warts; onion juice is said to eliminate athlete's foot; and onion can be used to combat indigestion. Also, according to folklore, onion restores male sexual potency.

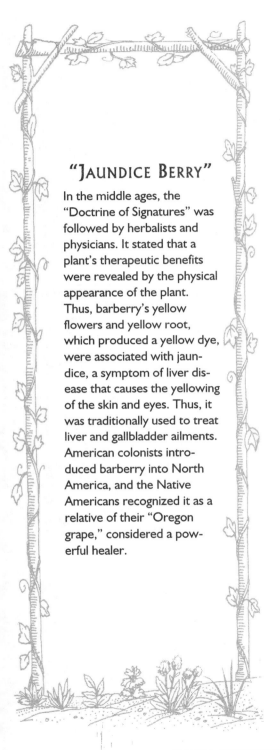

"Jaundice Berry"

In the middle ages, the "Doctrine of Signatures" was followed by herbalists and physicians. It stated that a plant's therapeutic benefits were revealed by the physical appearance of the plant. Thus, barberry's yellow flowers and yellow root, which produced a yellow dye, were associated with jaundice, a symptom of liver disease that causes the yellowing of the skin and eyes. Thus, it was traditionally used to treat liver and gallbladder ailments. American colonists introduced barberry into North America, and the Native Americans recognized it as a relative of their "Oregon grape," considered a powerful healer.

Contemporary herbalists recommend it as a sedative, antidepressant, and digestive stimulant, and to treat stress, bronchitis, indigestion, asthma, and infant colic. It is also used to promote sweating and for relaxing and restoring the nervous system. Science has proved Dioscorides correct by finding that balm contains polyphenols that fight infection-causing bacteria, including streptococci. It also contains eugenol, an anesthetic.

German researchers have discovered that balm oil—which is the source of the plant's pleasing fragrance—possesses tranquilizing properties, supporting the traditional use of the herb as a relaxant. They have also proved that balm relaxes the smooth-muscle tissue of the digestive tract, proof of its ancient use as a digestive aid. This same property can calm the uterus, another smooth muscle, which may explain its traditional use to ease menstrual cramps. However, it has also been recommended as a stimulant to promote menstruation and so should not be used by pregnant women. Nonpregnant women may use it to induce a period.

Dosage

Infusion of leaves: It is best made with fresh leaves harvested before the plant flowers. Use 2 teaspoons of leaves per cup of boiling water and steep 10 to 20 minutes. Drink up to 3 cups per day.

Tincture: This is stronger than the infusion and also best when made with fresh leaves. Use in small doses of 5 to 10 drops up to 3 times daily.

Compress: Soak a gauze pad in the infusion and apply to relieve painful swellings, especially around joints. Fresh leaves can be crushed and applied directly to a minor cut or wound.

Ointment: Commercially prepared ointments with balm can be used to repel insects; it can also be used on bites or on sores.

BARBERRY (*Berberis vulgaris*)

Common names: Berberry, jaundice berry, sowberry
Medicinal parts: Root bark, berries
Description: A deciduous shrub, barberry grows in the northeastern United States and in the western States. The root is yellow, and the leaves are oval. Small, yellow flowers appear

from April to June. Bright red, oblong berries ripen in August and September and should be eaten only when ripe.

Today barberry is primarily used as a decoction for gargling to treat sore throat. It is also drunk for diarrhea and constipation. Recent investigation has shown the berberine in barberry to have antibiotic properties, killing microorganisms that cause wound infections, diarrhea, dysentery, cholera, urinary tract infections, and vaginal yeast infections. It may also stimulate the immune system by strengthening the white blood cells. Additionally, it may also be helpful in reducing high blood pressure as it contains chemicals that enlarge blood vessels. However, although British researchers have isolated some substances that promote bile flow, its traditional use as a treatment for liver disease has not stood up to scientific investigation.

In Germany it is used to treat "pinkeye," or conjunctivitis, but commercial products for that use are not available here.

Barberry is a powerful herb and should be used cautiously in consultation with your doctor. Pregnant women should never take it because berberine stimulates the uterus.

Dosage

Decoction: Use $\frac{1}{2}$ teaspoon of powdered root bark per cup of water; boil for 15 to 30 minutes. Cool. Drink only 1 cup daily. It is bitter and can be sweetened with honey.

Compress: To treat conjunctivitis (pinkeye), soak a gauze pad in the infusion and apply to the closed eye.

BASIL *(Ocimum basilicum)*

Common names: Sweet basil, St. Josephwort
Medicinal parts: Leaves and flower tops
Description: An annual plant, it is cultivated as a kitchen herb but has been used for thousands of years as a medicinal herb. It has a lovely odor. A thin branch produces bushy stems 1 to 2 feet high at maturity, with toothed leaves. Flowers appear from June to September.

Basil's reputation as a healing herb has been in dispute for centuries. The Greeks and Romans reviled it, and the Italian folk

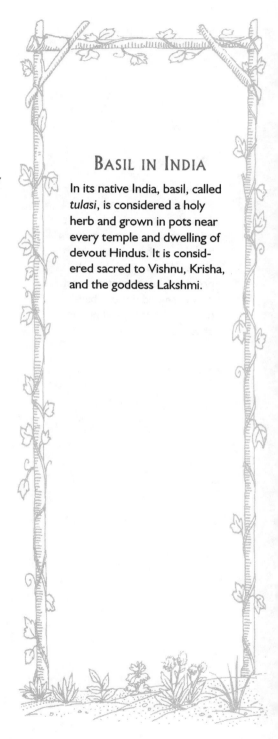

BASIL IN INDIA

In its native India, basil, called *tulasi*, is considered a holy herb and grown in pots near every temple and dwelling of devout Hindus. It is considered sacred to Vishnu, Krisha, and the goddess Lakshmi.

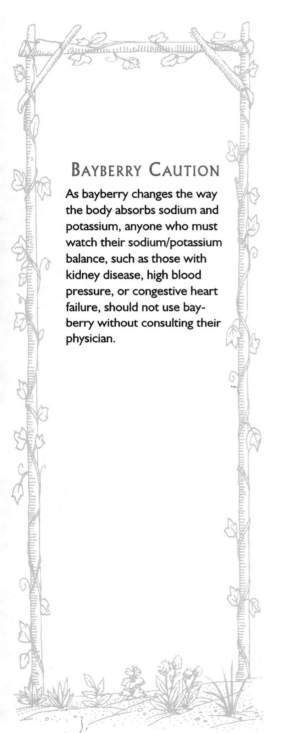

BAYBERRY CAUTION

As bayberry changes the way the body absorbs sodium and potassium, anyone who must watch their sodium/potassium balance, such as those with kidney disease, high blood pressure, or congestive heart failure, should not use bayberry without consulting their physician.

tradition associated it with love. Arab physicians defended it as a great healer, and the Chinese used it to treat stomach, kidney, and blood problems.

American herbalists today suggest it as a digestive aid and appetite stimulant and to promote milk in lactating women. Not just a delicious flavoring agent or the main component of pesto sauce, basil is an effective remedy for many digestive disorders such as stomach cramps and vomiting. The oil it contains kills intestinal parasites.

According to Louise Tenney, M.H., author of *Today's Herbal Health*, basil is useful for whooping cough and can help counteract insect stings or venomous snake bites.

Basil

Dosage

Dried herb: Mix 2 teaspoons of dried herbs with 1 cup of boiling water. Steep 10 minutes. Strain. Drink up to 3 cups daily.

BAYBERRY (*Myrica Cerrifera*)

Common names: Wax myrtle, candleberry tallow shrub
Medicinal part: Root bark
Description: Native to the United States from New Jersey to the Great Lakes and south to Florida and Texas, the bayberry tree is an evergreen that can reach 30 feet or more. Its dense, narrow toothed leaves are aromatic when crushed, and its yellow flowers, which appear in spring, produce nutlike fruits that are covered with the wax from which colonists made candles. The root bark is harvested when the plant is mature.

The early American colonists found the abundant bayberry tree a source for making fragrant candles, until they learned from the Choctaw Indians that the herb could be made into a decoction for treatment of fever. A 19th-century New England herbalist, Samuel A. Thomson, creator of some of the first patent medicines, said it produced "heat" within the body and recommended bayberry for respiratory ailments, in addition to

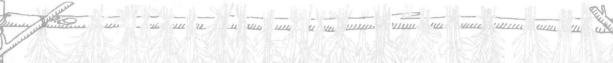

FERTILITY FEARS

Although Dr. Shealy advises women attempting to conceive to avoid turmeric, other fears about various herbs causing infertility have been put to rest. According to a July, 1999 article in *Prevention* magazine, a study from Loma Linda University School of Medicine in California created concerns—and lots of media attention—when it appeared to find that echinacea, St. John's wort, ginkgo, and saw palmetto could inhibit conception (in hamster eggs).

Varro E. Tyler, Ph.D., said in that article that the real problem seems to be the research. He states, "This study has more holes in it than a piece of Swiss cheese," and notes that in real life the active constituents of herbs must be absorbed into the bloodstream in order to have an effect. The article goes on to say that it is very unlikely that such levels would reach concentrations equal to the high levels (to which the hamster eggs were exposed) in this study. He speculates that any drug tested in this manner could "provoke similar problems," and goes on to state that, "echinacea, St. John's wort, ginkgo, and saw palmetto have been used by humans in millions of doses during recent years without a single negative fertility report."

fever. Then, unfortunately, it was forgotten as a medicinal, until the recent revival of interest in herbal remedies.

The root bark contains an antibiotic called myricitrin that is effective against a wide range of bacteria and protozoa, a finding that supports its traditional use as a specific for diarrhea and dysentery, as well as helping to reduce fever.

According to health writer Earl Mindell, bayberry is one of the oldest remedies for hemorrhoids, due no doubt to its powerful astringent qualities.

In India, the powdered root bark is combined with ginger to combat cholera, and it is considered to be a cleansing agent for the blood.

Dosage

Capsules: Take 1 to 3 daily or as recommended by the manufacturer.

Extract: Take 10 to 20 drops mixed with water or juice.

Decoction: Add 1 teaspoon of the powdered root bark to a pint of boiling water and steep 10 to 20 minutes. Cool. Drink up to 2 cups daily. It's bitter and very astringent. Its high tannin accounts for this; adding milk counteracts the tannin, which can irritate the stomach lining. If you have a history of stomach disorders, do not drink bayberry tea.

Mouthwash: Gargle with a liquid mixture according to directions given above to sooth sore or sensitive gums.

BILBERRY (*Vaccinium myrtillus*)

Common names: Black whortleberry, blueberry, burren myrtle, dyeberry, huckleberry, whortleberry, wineberry

Medicinal parts: Leaves, berries

Description: A shrubby perennial, bilberry grows in the sandy areas of the northern United States and in the woods and meadows of Europe. Although often called huckleberry, bilberry is more closely related to the cranberry.

Bilberry is an amazing dual-purpose herb that has been a well-known folk remedy for ages but has only recently again come to the attention of herbalists and those interested in alternative medicine.

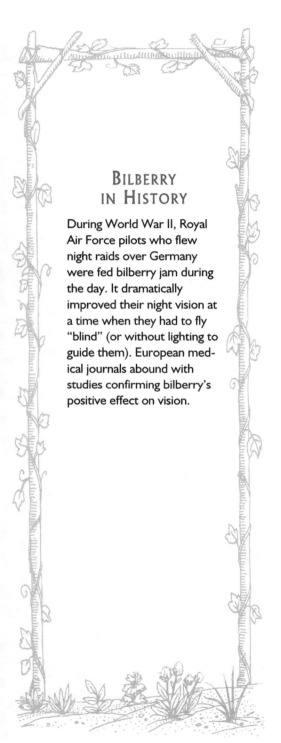

BILBERRY IN HISTORY

During World War II, Royal Air Force pilots who flew night raids over Germany were fed bilberry jam during the day. It dramatically improved their night vision at a time when they had to fly "blind" (or without lighting to guide them). European medical journals abound with studies confirming bilberry's positive effect on vision.

Its common use is for night blindness and to help preserve healthy eyesight, and it has been found to be beneficial in preventing the development of cataracts and to protect eyesight against damage caused by diabetes.

Bilberry's second use is for circulatory improvement. The herb helps to supply oxygen to the blood, thus feeding the capillaries and improving circulation by allowing more fluid and nutriments to pass through them.

Dosage

Capsules: Take 1 or 2 capsules twice daily, or follow the manufacturer's recommendations for dosage. *Do not* exceed the recommended amount, as the leaves can be poisonous if consumed over a long period of time. As with all herbs, they should be used only until the condition for which they are being taken has improved.

BLACK COHOSH (*Cimicifuga racemosa*)

Common names: Black snakeroot, bugbane, bugwort, rattleroot, rattleweed, richweed, squawroot

Medicinal part: Rootstock

Description: A native North American perennial, black cohosh is found on hillsides and in woods at higher elevations from Maine and Ontario to Wisconsin, Georgia, and Missouri. The rootstock is large, creeping, and knotty, producing a stem up to 9 feet high. It flowers from May to August.

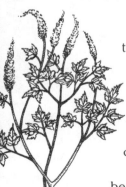

Black cohosh was used by Native Americans to reduce the pain and inflammation of rheumatism. It was also used to induce menstruation, relieve menstrual cramps, and to facilitate labor and aid delivery. Pregnant women should not use the herb until onset of labor, and then only under the supervision of their health care practitioner.

Today, has its traditional use for women has been proven by scientific studies. It is also recommended as a treatment for persistent coughs in cases of asthma, bronchitis, and whooping cough

Black Cohosh

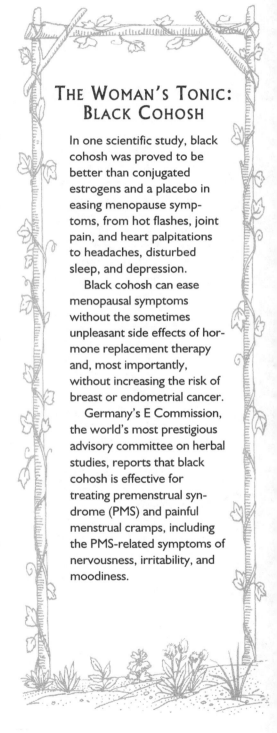

THE WOMAN'S TONIC: BLACK COHOSH

In one scientific study, black cohosh was proved to be better than conjugated estrogens and a placebo in easing menopause symptoms, from hot flashes, joint pain, and heart palpitations to headaches, disturbed sleep, and depression.

Black cohosh can ease menopausal symptoms without the sometimes unpleasant side effects of hormone replacement therapy and, most importantly, without increasing the risk of breast or endometrial cancer.

Germany's E Commission, the world's most prestigious advisory committee on herbal studies, reports that black cohosh is effective for treating premenstrual syndrome (PMS) and painful menstrual cramps, including the PMS-related symptoms of nervousness, irritability, and moodiness.

CAYENNE THEN AND NOW

The red hot chili known as cayenne was brought to the West in 1548 from its native India. The 16th-century herbalist John Gerard called it "extreme hot and dry, even in the fourth degree," and recommended it for scrofula, commonly known as the "King's Evil." Called "Ginnie pepper," cayenne was used by 19th-century "physiomedicalists" for chills, rheumatism, and depression.

It is used today as a potent stimulant for the whole body and considered a tonic for the nervous system. Hot herbs are supposed to increase metabolism rate, and cayenne may help with weight loss. Recently, research has suggested that cayenne can ease the severe pain of shingles and migraines. It is readily available in powered form or as a bottled hot sauce.

because of its ability to relieve muscle spasms. It relaxes bronchial tubes, quelling the urge to cough, and allows the entire body to relax.

Dosage

Capsules: Take 1 to 3 capsules daily, according to the manufacturer's instructions, or 40 milligrams daily.

Tincture: Take 1 teaspoon total per day.

Infusion: Make a tea by pouring 3 cups of boiling water over 1 tablespoon of the dried root and steep, covered, for 10 minutes. Strain. Drink 3 cups daily.

Poultice: Soak a clean cloth in the infusion for use against inflammation. Apply to affected area several times daily.

Cough syrup: Commercial preparations of black cohosh cough syrup are available through health food stores or mail order suppliers. Follow directions given by manufacturer.

CARAWAY (Carum carvi)

Common name: Generally called caraway; also carum

Medicinal part: Fruit ("seeds")

Description: A feathery-leafed biennial that can reach 2 feet, caraway's early summer umbrella-like clusters of tiny white flowers become its fruit, which we call seeds.

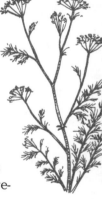

Caraway

Primarily known as a flavoring agent for breads and candy, caraway seeds have been used since prehistoric times and were recommended for digestive upsets in the Papyrus Ebers written in Egypt c. 1500 B.C.E., one of the world's oldest surviving medical documents.

Only a few herbs are still used today as they were in ancient times, and caraway is one of these rare cases. Down through the ages, they have been taken for indigestion and flatulence and given to infants for colic. The only other traditional use for caraway is for women's health—to ease menstrual cramps, increase menstrual flow, and promote milk in nursing mothers.

Dosage

Seeds (fresh or dried): Chew a teaspoonful of whole seeds or mix into any food.

Infusion: Crush 2 to 3 teaspoons of seeds per cup of boiling water. Steep 10 to 20 minutes and drink up to 3 cups daily. Dilute infusion for infant colic.

CHAMOMILE *(Matricaria chamomilla; Anthemis nobilis)*

Common names: Ground apple, whig plant, matricaria
Medicinal parts: Flowers
Description: Extremely aromatic, common chamomile (called "Roman") is cultivated in gardens and can be found in fields growing wild. It flowers during June and July. Flowers should be quickly dried to retain their pungent scent.

The Greeks called chamomile "ground apple" for its fragrance; to the Anglo–Saxons, it was maythen, one of nine sacred herbs that the Norse god, Woden, gave to humans.

Chamomile is today one of the best-selling herbs. As a tea, it is favored for its relaxing properties as well as its apple-like aroma and is known to soothe the nerves and restore vitality.

Contemporary herbalists also recommend chamomile for external use to speed the healing of wounds and treat inflammation. Internally, it is given for fever, digestive upsets, anxiety, and insomnia.

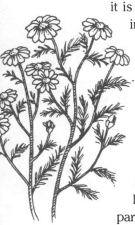

Chamomile

The German chamomile is commonly known as "matricaria," a reference to its antispasmodic properties, which have made it an age-old herb used to ease menstrual cramps. In Germany, where herbal healing is mainstream and not considered "alternative," chamomile is so popular that it is called *alles zutraut*, or all-purpose. Long used to prevent wound infection, only recently did British researchers discover that chamomile stimulates the immune system's white blood cells. It's particularly recommended for use at the onset of a cold or the flu and its warming and soothing properties promote sleep, the greatest curative of all.

ARE YOU A CHAMOMILLA TYPE?

Chamomile is also prepared as a homeopathic remedy, called chamomilla. The person most likely to benefit from taking chamomilla is impulsive, restless, sensitive—wears her emotions on her sleeve, so to speak. The chamomilla type suffers acutely from pain but often uses denial as a defense, refusing help, even when symptoms are serious.

To determine if you're a chamomilla type, check the following characteristics that apply to you:

- Anger makes you feel bad.
- Getting along with others is a problem for you.
- You suffer from irritability.
- Indecisiveness causes you to be argumentative.
- Wind and heat bother you excessively.

If you checked three or more of the above items, chamomilla may help relieve your suffering.

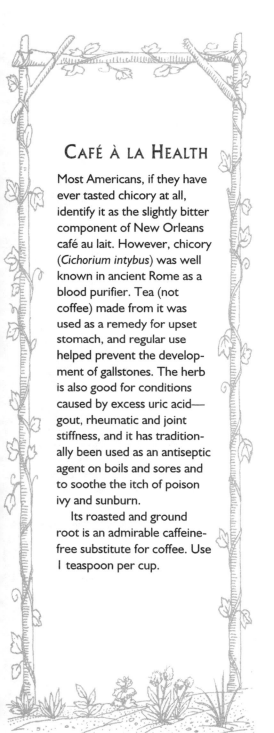

CAFÉ À LA HEALTH

Most Americans, if they have ever tasted chicory at all, identify it as the slightly bitter component of New Orleans café au lait. However, chicory (*Cichorium intybus*) was well known in ancient Rome as a blood purifier. Tea (not coffee) made from it was used as a remedy for upset stomach, and regular use helped prevent the development of gallstones. The herb is also good for conditions caused by excess uric acid— gout, rheumatic and joint stiffness, and it has traditionally been used as an antiseptic agent on boils and sores and to soothe the itch of poison ivy and sunburn.

Its roasted and ground root is an admirable caffeine-free substitute for coffee. Use 1 teaspoon per cup.

Generally speaking, chamomile is one of the safest herbs available. However, if you are allergic to ragweed or have ever suffered anaphylactic shock, avoid this herb.

Dosage

Tea: Chamomile tea bags are available in health food stores and some supermarkets. It can be obtained in bulk from health food stores. Steep a tea bag in a cup of boiling water for 5 minutes, or make an infusion from 2 or 3 teaspoons of the bulk herb. Drink a cup or two for relaxation, or at night to promote sleep.

The infusion can also be used as a mouthwash to heal inflamed gums or mouth sores. Dilute it for infant colic. For wounds and abrasions, soak a gauze pad in the infusion and apply it to the afflicted part.

COMFREY (*Symphytum oficinale*)

Common names: Bruisewort, knitbone, salsify, wallwort
Medicinal parts: Roots and leaves
Description: Common in moist meadows and other damp places in the United Sates and Europe, comfrey is a perennial with a root that contains a glutinous juice. The tongue-shaped leaves lie on the ground. Flowers appear from May to August.

Although generations of healers have treated skin wounds with comfrey successfully, they never knew why or how it worked. Today, we know comfrey contains allantoin, which helps stimulate the growth of new cells. Once commonly taken internally, its internal use is currently controversial. Some believe it should never be ingested, because it contains potential cancer-causing components. When taken in large amounts, it has been shown to cause liver cancer. However, Britain's National Institute of Medical Herbalists states flatly that "no man, woman, or child has been recorded as suffering toxic effects from taking [recommended doses] of comfrey leaf or root as medicine." And cancer authority Bruce Ames, Ph.D., chairman of the biochemistry department at the University of California at Berkeley, estimated that a cup of comfrey tea poses about the same cancer risk as does a peanut butter sandwich—peanut butter contain

CAFFEINE IN PLANTS

Following are seven caffeine-containing plants more widely used by humans than all other herbal remedies combined:

- **Coffee.** Coffee contains 1 to 2 percent caffeine
- **Tea.** Depending on the method of preparation and the varieties of the cultivated plant, the caffeine content of tea varies from less than 1 percent to more than 4 percent.
- **Green tea.** Green tea is now becoming a popular beverage because of its antioxidant properties. Its caffeine content also varies, but drinking it provides health benefits.
- **Kola (Cola or Kolanuts).** It is from kola that our popular cola drinks originally got their name. Typically, kola contains about 3 percent caffeine.
- **Cacao (Cocoa).** Not to be confused with coca, the source of cocaine, or coconut, the fruit of a palm tree, cacao yields chocolate. It contains between 0.07 and 0.36 percent caffeine and should not be given to children under three years of age.
- **Guarana.** Native to Brazil and Uruguay, guarana has a high caffeine content of from 2.5 to 5 percent, averaging 3.5 percent. Today it is an ingredient in carbonated sodas marketed by the Coca-Cola Company in Brazil and the Pepsi-Cola Company in the United States.
- **Maté.** Another South American herb, maté is made into a tea-like drink purported to increase energy and provide stamina. Containing up to 2 percent caffeine, depending on the strength of the brew.

Below is a guideline for approximate amounts of caffeine in commonly used foods and beverages:

Coffee, brewed from ground beans—6 oz.	100 mg.
Coffee, instant—6 oz.	65 mg.
Tea, brewed from whole leaves—6 oz.	10–50 mg.
Cola, can or bottle—12 oz.	50 mg.
Cocoa, breakfast type—6 oz.	13 mg.
Cocoa, as milk chocolate bar—1 oz.	6 mg
Guarana, tablet or capsule—800 mg.	30 mg.
Maté, brewed as tea—6 oz.	25–50 mg.
Caffeine tablet, proprietary product	100–200 mg.

CHIVES—THE HERBAL EXORCIST

In the Middle Ages, chives were believed to drive away evil spirits and cure melancholy. Bundles of the herb were hung from rafters and bedposts. Today, we know that chives and chive flowers are high in vitamin C, folic acid, potassium, calcium, and blood-building iron; and that they stimulate the appetite and promote good digestion, reduce flatulence, and prevent bad breath. Even better, recent scientific research shows that chives, when eaten regularly, may help to lower blood cholesterol levels. Because of their high vitamin C content, they can help prevent colds or speed recovery from a cold; the sulfurous compounds in them are natural expectorants. Best used fresh, they are easy to grow in pots at home.

～～

Snip chives with kitchen scissors to prevent loss of their essential oils. Cut them only when the long slender leaves reach about 6 inches in height; harvest often.

traces of the natural carcinogen aflatoxin. Since the FDA lists comfrey as an herb of "undefined safety," it should be taken with caution and the advice of a medical professional or not ingested.

CRANBERRY (*Vaccinium macrocarpon, Oxycoccus quadripetalus*)

Common name: Cranberry

Medicinal parts: Juice from the berries, whole berries

Description: Cranberries grow in bogs from Alaska to Tennessee and are a main crop in Maine. The bright red small berry fruit is harvested in fall.

Cranberry

Traditionally made into a sauce to serve with the Thanksgiving turkey, the common cranberry has a powerful medicinal use as an agent against urinary infection and cystitis. Doctors routinely advise their patients troubled with these afflictions to drink cranberry juice, and it is listed as an effective remedy in the *United States Pharmacopoeia*, the official United States list of approved drugs.

The problem with commercially produced cranberry juice "cocktail" generally purchased in supermarkets is that it is more water and sugar than actual cranberry juice. To get enough of the pure juice, it's necessary to drink a large quantity—as much as a quart a day, which is often not practical. Fortunately, health food stores carry a bottled pure cranberry juice concentrate that can be diluted at home to suit one's own taste. Personally, I enjoy its natural tartness, but if you find it too sour, you can sweeten it as you please. Of course, if you use sugar or honey, you are adding calories. One good sweetener is an infusion made from licorice root (which does not taste like the licorice candy you know from childhood—that taste comes not from licorice but from anise seeds). Another solution is to mix the pure cranberry juice with unprocessed apple juice that is sugar-free, or buy a commercial brand of

Chives

cranberry juice sweetened naturally with apple and grape juices. Encapsulated dried berries are also effective for active urinary infections. You can also munch on the new dried cranberries, sometimes called "craisins" for their similarity to raisins.

Once a urinary infection has been cleared up, continue to drink a glass of pure cranberry juice daily as a preventative against future infection, especially if you are a sexually active woman who is prone to cystitis.

DANDELION (*Taraxacum officinale*)

Common names: Puffball, cankerwort, lion's tooth, wild endive, white endive.

Medicinal parts: Leaves and root.

Description: This perennial plant, often the bane of those who yearn for perfectly manicured lawns, is found just about everywhere. It sends up, from a milky taproot, one or more naked flower stems, each of which is topped by a single yellow flower. The familiar "puffball" is a fluffy globular cluster of individual seeds cleverly fitted with a parachute-like tuft that enables it to travel far and wide on the wind.

For a common plant that is vilified by lawn lovers everywhere, who will go to great length to destroy it in their yards, dandelion has remarkable healing properties. And as it's so readily available— ubiquitous in North America—that it is not better appreciated is a shame.

Actually, there are literally hundreds of subspecies of dandelion, which vary in appearance from one another to the extent that they can only be recognized by botanists.

As a healing plant, dandelion is a natural diuretic and digestive aid, a laxative and stomach remedy, a promoter of healthy circulation, and a blood vessel cleanser and strengthener. Rich in potassium, which works with sodium to regulate the body's mineral and fluid balance, dandelion enhances liver and gallbladder function. Traditional herbalists use it to treat jaundice—as it is rich in lecithin, a substance researchers think protects against cirrhosis of the liver; this old remedy has modern support.

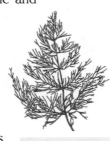

Dill

CAN ECHINACEA HELP CURE CANCER?

An article in the *Journal of Medical Chemistry* reported that an extract made from echinacea was shown to inhibit tumor growth in rats. Further studies are needed, but echinacea already shows promise as an anticancer treatment.

Echinacea's immune-boosting effect may help cancer patients undergoing radiation therapy by protecting the white blood cells and lessen the chance of secondary infection. Patients in radiation therapy would be well advised to discuss using echinacea with their doctors.

∽

Don't wait until cold and flu season arrives before getting a supply of echinacea. It's an extremely popular remedy and even well-stocked health food stores can run short during cold and flu season. It's a good idea to keep a bottle on hand at all times—there's really nothing nastier than a bad *summer* cold or out-of-season flu.

As if those properties were not sufficient, this despised little plant can also cure rheumatism and soothe badly affected arthritic joints. The juice of the broken stem will remove warts when applied and allowed to dry for three days in a row. And it's a bracing tonic for fatigue!

Dandelion

According to herbalist Varro E. Tyler, Ph.D., dandelion is useful in treating fungus infections, external and internal malignant growths, ulceration of the urinary passages, and obstructions of the liver, gallbladder, and spleen. He further states that it makes a fine wine and a great beer, as well as an excellent coffee substitute. Dandelion wine was a staple of homemade comestibles in earlier times.

Bloating, breast tenderness, swelling of the hands and feet, and weight gain are the second most common collection of PMS symptoms. Kidney hormones, which control diuresis and salt retention, are considered responsible for the condition. For relief, dandelion can help. Double the suggested dosages for the 10 days before you expect your period to begin.

If you have an abundance of dandelions in your yard, pick them and dry your own leaves. Or for a spring tonic, press the juice from the stems with an electric juicer. Mix a teaspoon of the juice in 4 ounces of milk and drink.

Dosage

Capsules: Take 1 to 3 daily, or follow directions on the manufacturer's label.

Extract: Take 10 to 30 drops in a liquid daily.

Fresh stems: Break them open and use to treat warts.

Fresh roots: Bring water to boil and add root. Let steep for 15 minutes to make a tea.

Fresh leaves: Use in salads or as a garnish. Just make sure they have not been sprayed with pesticides.

THE ORIGINAL "SNAKE OIL"

Echinacea was the Plains Indians' primary medicine. It was first used as a remedy for snakebite, skin wounds, and the bites and stings of insects, poisonous and otherwise. As a tea, it was used to treat all manner of ailments, from painful teeth and gums to colds, arthritis, smallpox, measles, and mumps.

Pronounced eh-kin-AY-sha. Plains settlers used the plant as a popular folk remedy until 1870, when a patent medicine purveyor, Dr. H. C. F. Meyer of Pawnee City, Nebraska, included it as an ingredient in his "Meyer's Blood Purifier," which he promoted as an "absolute cure" for snakebite and a wide range of other ailments. Thus it was that patent medicines were dubbed "snake oil" by those who listened to the often hyperbolic harangues of their salesmen. To prove his claims, Dr. Meyer sent off a sample to John Uri Lloyd, professor at the Eclectic Medical Institute in Cincinnati, later president of the American Pharmaceutical Association. Lloyd identified the plant as echinacea but dismissed Meyer's claims as "hogwash."

However, later Lloyd accepted that echinacea was useful in treating wounds, venomous bites and stings, blood poisoning, diphtheria, meningitis, measles, chicken pox, scarlet fever, influenza, syphilis, and gangrene. His enthusiasm was commercial as well as professional, and the Lloyd Brothers Pharmacists developed many products made from echinacea that were best-selling medicines from the 1890s well into the 1920s, during which time tincture of echinacea was as common in medicine cabinets as aspirin is today.

ECHINACEA EVERY DAY?

Germany's Commission E, the only government organization that seriously studies and closely monitors the use and effectiveness of herbal remedies, suggests limiting the use of oral consumption of echinacea to a maximum of 8 weeks in succession. However, herbal expert Varro E. Tyler, Ph.D. and herbal advisor to *Prevention* magazine, states that there is no proof that continued use lessens echinacea's effectiveness or causes any deleterious effects.

Nonetheless, Dr. Tyler agrees with the German advice on the principle that any herbal products should be taken only when needed. However, he says that "If you want to use it on a more regular basis, go ahead." The choice is yours.

ECHINACEA (*Echinacea angustifolia, E.*)

Common names: Purple coneflower, black samson, rudbeckia, Missouri snakeroot

Medicinal part: Root (rhizome)

Description: This perennial plant is native to the United States and grows from the prairie states northward to Pennsylvania. It is one of the most common wildflowers found in the state of Texas. Its pinkish flower petals droop down from a center of spiky yellow to gold stamen, possibly accounting for its common name of "purple coneflower." It is easy to recognize.

Echinacea

Today, however, the more specific designation, narrow-leafed echinacea, is used to describe the plant, a member of the daisy family. Nine known species of echinacea grow in the United States. In addition to *E. angustifolia*, there is *Echinacea pallida*, known as pale-flowered echinacea, and *Echinacea purpurea,* the commonly cultivated garden variety. All of these are used in commercial echinacea products and *E. purpurea* is the most common variety used in commercial preparations.

Unfortunately, echinacea waned in popularity as the "Eclectic" physicians lost ground to the "regular" allopathic physicians, who preferred to rely on synthetic pharmaceutical drugs. As early as 1909, the *Journal of the American Medical Association* denounced echinacea as useless and by the 1930s, when antibiotics became available, it was relegated to the history books.

That is, until the herbal renaissance begun during the 1970s sparked interest in this herb's many excellent healing properties, especially its positive effect on the immune system. We now know from many studies that echinacea prevents formation of hyaluronidase, an enzyme that destroys the natural barrier between healthy tissue and invading pathogenic organisms. It is especially useful against viruses.

As many types of flu and some colds are caused by viruses, echinacea is Mother Nature's most powerful agent for fighting them. Widely used in Europe, it works by giving the immune system a jump-start, a powerful boost that works quickly, reducing symptoms while your immune system gets to work clearing out the invaders. A 1978 study in *Planta Medica* showed that an extract from the root of echinacea destroyed herpes viruses as well as influenza viruses. European studies also show that echinacea lessens the severity of colds and flu and speeds recovery, especially when taken at the onset of symptoms.

It has also proved beneficial in treating the annoying and persistent fungal yeast infection known as candida that often troubles women. Used in combination with an antifungal cream, echinacea extract served to prevent recurrence of candida symptoms in patients tested. As a skin ointment, echinacea has been successfully used to treat psoriasis and eczema.

Dosage

Capsules or tablets: Buy standardized preparations made from the roots or tops of the species *Echinacea angustifolia, E. pallida*, or *E. purpurea.* Use them individually and not in a product that combines echinacea with other herbs. Follow the manufacturer's directions for amount to use.

Extract: Mix 15 to 30 drops of commercially prepared tincture in any liquid and drink 3 times daily until symptoms are gone.

EPHEDRA *(Ephedra sinica)*

Common name: Ma huang
Medicinal parts: Stems, root
Description: Not an ordinary garden herb, ephedra is an odd-looking, botanically primitive shrub. Almost leafless, it resembles horsetail. The tough, jointed, barkless stems produce small scale-like leaves. Tiny yellow-green flowers appear in summer, and seeds develop in cone-shaped pods.

Ephedra is considered to be the world's oldest medicine, part of an herbal healing tradition dating back over 5000 years. Its origins in Chinese medicine are unknown, but authorities believe that Chinese physicians began prescribing *ma huang* for colds and other respiratory problems (such as asthma and bronchial infections) around the year 3000 B.C.E. The Indian and Pakistani varieties of the herb have been used about as long.

Though *ma huang* has had a long history, its active constituent, ephedrine, was not isolated until 1887 by Japanese

GYPSY GIFT

Since time immemorial, gypsies have used the berry of the elderberry tree as a remedy for colds, influenza, and neuralgia. The traditional gypsy formula for coughs and bronchial infections called for elderberry juice to be pressed from the tree's berries and boiled, together with crab apple juice and honey, to make a syrup. Today, you can prepare an effective remedy from store-bought elderberry tea and add your own honey and a bit of lemon.

Gypsies also made elderberry into a salve or ointment to treat skin inflammations, eczema, and dry skin. It's available in ointment form at health food stores today.

chemist N. Nagai. And it was not until 1924 that another Asian researcher, K. K. Chen, at Peking Union Medical College, published a series of papers on the pharmacological properties of the herb. From the late 1920s through the 1940s, ephedrine was used in decongestant products for colds and hay fever, and, in an inhalant form, was the drug of choice for asthma sufferers. Eventually, it was replaced by a close chemical substitute, pseudoephedrine, the active ingredient in many over-the-counter cold and allergy preparations (e.g., Sudafed).

When used as a stimulant, *ma huang* is more powerful than caffeine but less potent than amphetamine, stimulating the heart and increasing blood pressure and metabolic rate. It has recently come under controversy for these side effects, especially when used in products marketed to teens and youth as a legal "high." Genuine *ma huang*, and products containing it, should be used with caution when ingested and preferably under the supervision of a health care professional.

Dosage

Tea: Use twigs or the dried powdered herb to make an infusion. One teaspoon of powdered *ma huang* per cup of water will make an average strength decoction of which you can drink up to 2 cups per day.

Capsules or tablets: These are prepared commercially. Follow package directions *exactly* to avoid an overdose. Never give to children without consulting a pediatrician.

FEVERFEW (*Chrysanthemum parthenium*)

Common names: Featherfew, febrifuge plant
Medicinal parts: The entire herb
Description: A perennial, feverfew can reach 3 feet in height and produces pretty daisylike flowers. Mostly it is cultivated, but it can be found along roadsides and wood borders from Quebec to Ohio and south to Maryland and Missouri, and in California. It flowers in June and July.

A legendary herb since the time of Dioscorides (78 C.E.), it was used especially for the treatment of

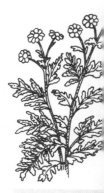

Feverfew

MORMON TEA

When the members of the Church of Latter-Day Saints reached Utah in 1847, Native Americans introduced them to the American form of ephedra. They found it made a pleasantly piney-flavored stimulating drink, which they used as a substitute for the coffee and tea forbidden to Mormons.

~

EVENING PRIMROSE STUDY

Swedish studies, though preliminary, are relating evening primrose oil to an antioxidant that counteracts the formation of free radicals, which are especially active in the aging process.

~

EUCALYPTUS TIP

Oil of eucalyptus is a wonderful way to clear a stuffy nose and a foggy head. Just a sniff or two is all it takes. And a few drops in boiling water make a good steam inhalant.

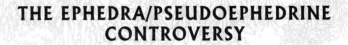

THE EPHEDRA/PSEUDOEPHEDRINE CONTROVERSY

The issue of ephedra's safety remains unresolved. Mainstream medical researchers claim that the commercial chemical preparation pseudoephedrine is safer than the herbal ephedra. Many herbalists agree, but they insist that when the *entire* plant is used, no question of safety arises. In *Herbal Medicine for Everyone*, British herbalist Michael McIntry writes that "pure ephedrine markedly raises blood pressure . . . . But the whole plant actually reduces blood pressure." And Rudolph Fritz Weiss, M.D., a German medical herbalist, maintains that the whole plant has "certain advantages [over pseudoephedrine]" because "it is better tolerated, causing fewer heart symptoms such as palpitations." Certainly, anyone with high blood pressure should consult a physician before using any ephedra product.

As it is such a powerful stimulant, ephedra should not be taken by people with sleep problems, nor should it be ingested late in the day.

Competitive athletes tend to favor its use, but they should be extremely careful with it. Because of its possible misuse, it is on the list of substances banned by the United States Olympic Committee.

Young people should avoid it altogether unless it is prescribed by their doctor.

migraine headaches but also for menstrual irregularities, stomach complaints, and particularly fever. In fact, its common name is a corruption of the Latin word *febrifugia,* which means "fever reducer." Despite this long history, feverfew fell into disuse until the late 1970s, when persons afflicted with painful and debilitating migraines were unable to find relief through conventional allopathic means. As they turned to alternatives, feverfew was resurrected and is now "hot" as recent studies have shown just how effective it is in preventing migraine headaches.

The return of feverfew was sparked in 1978, when a woman cured herself of migraines with feverfew leaves and the story was reported in British newspapers. As a result, serious medical researchers decided to study the herb. In 1985, *Lancet,* the prestigious British medical journal, published an article that reported that extracts of feverfew inhibited the release of two substances considered to bring on migraine attacks—serotonin from platelets and prostaglandin from white blood cells. And in 1988, *Lancet* published a report of a carefully designed study that proved the herb's power to prevent migraine headaches and/or lessen the severity of the attack. This information came as no surprise to herbalists. However, it is important to note that feverfew does not actually *cure* migraine; it only helps prevent or lessen it. Luckily for migraine sufferers, who may end up taking it for years, long-term use has not been shown to be a problem, although more research is needed to determine long-term effects, if any. It can take several months of regular use for feverfew to work, so if you suffer from migraines, don't get discouraged.

Dosage

Fresh leaves: Eat 1 large leaf daily as a prophylactic against migraine headaches.

Capsules or tablets: As feverfew is bitter as an infusion, or when chewing the fresh leaves, most people will prefer capsules or tablets taken orally. When buying these commercially prepared products, be sure to read the label; some brands contain only trace amounts of the pure herb.

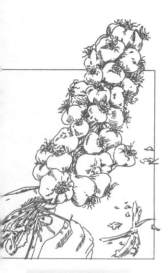

Garlic

GARLIC (*Allium sativum*)

Common name: None

Medicinal part: Bulb

Description: So common is this herb it hardly needs describing. A perennial widely cultivated, it is one of the most common herbs, the bulb consisting of individual "cloves" that easily break off.

Garlic may be the oldest medicinal herb known to humans. There are those who think it is the wonder drug of the herbal pharmacy, so many and varied are the worldwide applications of this herb and its relatives; onions, leeks, and shallots are well-known members of the lily family.

Much folkloric use of garlic as a medicinal herb has claimed it useful for everything from cancer and tuberculosis to hemorrhoids and even athlete's foot. Modern usage is primarily for treating atherosclerosis and hypertension. It can also be a powerful antibacterial agent, but only when chopped, mashed, or ground—which brings on garlic's significant drawback, that is, its pungent odor.

Garlic has been extensively investigated in modern times and is at least as potent as aspirin for use in prevention of blood clots that can trigger heart attack. Dutch researchers have published a detailed analysis of all the clinical studies on garlic's effects regarding various cardiovascular risk factors. Their conclusion is that in regard to fresh garlic, claims for beneficial effects on blood cholesterol levels, fibrinolytic activity, and platelet aggregation are valid. However, to gain these positive effects garlic must be eaten in fairly large quantities—5 to 25 average-sized cloves daily depending on body weight.

Other forms of garlic, such as freeze-dried capsules or deodorized or aged forms made into tablets or capsules may not be as effective as the fresh garlic. However, of these, the aged, odorless capsule is the favored form.

For maximum ease in preparing garlic for home consumption, invest in a garlic peeler and a garlic press. Since garlic is best

RUSSIAN PENICILLIN

Louis Pasteur, the famous French biologist, put a few garlic cloves in a Petri dish full of bacteria and, to his amazement, discovered that garlic could kill these deadly microorganisms. As a result of his discovery, when during World War I Russia's enormous number of casualties totally depleted its supply of antibiotics, Russian army physicians substituted garlic as a treatment for infected wounds, which earned it the sobriquet "Russian penicillin." And, in the 1950s, Dr. Albert Schweitzer used garlic to treat the African scourges of cholera, typhus, and amebic dysentery.

GINGER IN HISTORY

Ginger was probably one of the spices indigenous to the Orient to be imported to the great harbor city of Alexandria in Egypt, from which it went to Greece and Rome before the first century C.E. Dioscorides and Pliny mention ginger, and it appears in a recipe book by Apicius written at the height of Rome's luxurious days of glory.

Then worth its weight in gold, ginger could only be afforded by the rich. Known as *singabera*, its Sanskrit name, the root was cultivated in China and India from remote times. Legend has it that it was introduced into the western hemisphere by Francisco de Mendoca in the 16th century. Records of ginger shipments from Santo Domingo go back as far as 1585 and today, Jamaica, in the British West Indies, is the largest supplier of this popular herb.

when fresh (sprouted garlic is bitter), a special terra cotta storage pot for garlic is recommended.

Dosage

Fresh: Incorporate fresh garlic into salads by chopping, crushing, or putting through a garlic press (2 or 3 cloves a day is optimum).

Cooked: Sautéing 2 or 3 garlic cloves that have been mashed or chopped in a bit of oil will help eliminate the typical "garlic breath" and aftertaste. Be careful not to brown them, or they will become bitter. Whole garlic bulbs can be roasted in the oven and the individual cloves squeezed out onto bread or toast as a creamy spread. Long cooking eliminates garlic taste altogether.

Capsules: Take 1 to 3 capsules daily, or follow the label directions.

Tablets: Enteric-coated tablets of prepared garlic are now available commercially and appear to be a suitable and odor-free alternative to fresh garlic.

GINGER (*Zingiber officinale*)

Common names: Jamaica ginger, African ginger, Cochin ginger

Medicinal part: Root (technically, a rhizome)

Description: A perennial indigenous to tropical Asia, ginger is cultivated in other tropical areas, especially Jamaica. Its aromatic, branched rootstock is fibrous, juicy, and buff-colored.

Ginger's most frequent use is for nausea and upset stomach or stomach cramps. The Chinese have used ginger for 2000 years, and the Japanese serve ginger slices between courses to aid digestion. It is also a curative for motion sickness and dizziness, working better than the drug Dramamine, according to a study published in *Lancet*, a British medical journal.

Ginger

G IS FOR GREENS WITH
GARLIC ARE GOOD FOR YOU

A good way to work garlic into your diet is to cook with it. Combine garlic with super-nutritious greens using the easy stir-fry method. First, peel and mince some garlic cloves (the more the better!). Then, sauté in oil for about a minute. (Don't let the garlic brown, or it will become bitter.) Add the torn or sliced greens, prepared as indicated in the chart below, and cook only until tender; remove from heat while still bright green. Times given are approximate.

TYPE OF GREENS	PRECOOK PREPARATION	FRYING TIME
Beet greens	Rinse, pat dry	5 minutes
Bok choy	Rinse, remove thick stems, tear or slice leaves	5 minutes
Broccoli rabe	Rinse, remove thick stems, blanch 5 minutes, squeeze	5 minutes
Curly endive	Rinse, remove inner stems, tear or slice thinly	5 minutes
Collard greens	Rinse, cut out center stems, cut leaves into 1-inch pieces, blanch 3 minutes, squeeze	5 minutes
Dandelion greens	Rinse (twice if gathered wild), blanch 3 minutes	3 minutes
Escarole	Discard outer leaves, rinse, dry, tear or chop leaves	3 minutes
Kale	Cut out center rib, rinse, blanch 5 minutes, squeeze	5 minutes
Mustard greens	Rinse, discard center ribs, blanch 3 minutes, squeeze	5 minutes
Chinese cabbage	Rinse, slice, pat dry	3 minutes
Spinach	Rinse thoroughly, pat dry	2 minutes
Swiss chard	Rinse, discard stems, slice leaves, pat dry	3 minutes
Watercress	Rinse, remove stems	1 minute

Note: To blanch greens, drop them in boiling water for the time indicated; then, drain thoroughly and squeeze dry before frying. Be careful with blanched greens; if they are wet, the oil may splatter.

An excellent herb for fighting off colds and flu, ginger helps the respiratory system by removing congestion and easing aches and pains. In his recent book, *The Arthritis Bible,* health writer Craig Weathersby states that ginger, when used in sufficient quantities for a sufficient length of time, will aid arthritis sufferers.

Dosage

Capsules: This is the most common form for taking ginger medicinally. Capsules usually contain 500 milligrams of the powdered herb; 2 to 4 capsules daily is recommended.

Tea: A ginger tea can be brewed by steeping the fresh root—chopped or grated—in boiling water for 10 minutes. Drink plain or sweeten to taste.

Ginger ale: Commercial ginger ale, provided it is not artificially flavored, will help to settle the stomach. A 12-ounce glass is recommended—sip or drink as desired. Try adding some brewed ginger tea to your ginger ale to strengthen it; or add plain carbonated water to ginger tea to make a fizzy drink.

GINKGO *(Ginkgo biloba)*

Common name: Maidenhair tree
Medicinal part: Leaves
Description: A deciduous conifer with separate male and female forms. Introduced into Europe from the Far East in 1730, it became popular as an ornamental. Ginkgo trees, which can reach 100 feet with a 20-foot diameter, can be grown throughout much of the United States.

Ginkgo

Ginkgo biloba has recently come into immense popularity as an aid to memory. Used in China for thousands of years, extracts from the tree's leaves are today the source of an herbal remedy that is big news. In a recent study published in the *Journal of the American Medical Association,* researchers confirmed what earlier European research had already surmised: that people who take the ginko extract for mild to severe dementia may improve both their ability to remember and to interact socially.

UÑA DE GATO

Spanish for "cat's claw," this tropical member of the madder family grows a root that can be as large as a watermelon. The variety of ailments and applications that cat's claw is used for today, including arthritis, asthma, cancer, gastritis, and inflammation, is much the same as it was traditionally. Alexander G. Schauss, Ph.D., who has done extensive research on cat's claw, a Latin American botanical, quoted in the 1997 issue of *Better Nutrition* magazine, says of Latin America:

[It is] "certainly one of the last areas to be explored in terms of botanicals. It's an issue of ethnocentricity. In this country, most of our research on botanicals is on European herbs. Besides cat's claw there are probably countless other Latin American botanicals which still need to be explored, so I expect to see much more about Latin American herbs in the future."

The leaves of the ginkgo contain the active constituents ginkgo flavone glycosides and terpene lactones, the extract of which can be used to treat poor circulation in the legs as well as memory and cognitive problems. It is also possible that ginkgo may aid men who suffer from impotence induced by taking antidepressant medications.

Though ginkgo has no history in Western herbal lore, European herbalists and mainstream physicians are so enthusiastic about its healing properties for a variety of ailments that it is among Europe's most widely used herbal remedies, with sales totaling $500 million a year.

Of botanicals used to treat conditions common in older people, ginkgo biloba is one of the most popular, usually as a memory enhancer. A five-year study to determine if ginkgo can prevent dementia in older people or enhance memory in otherwise healthy people has been undertaken by the NIH Center for Complementary and Alternative Medicine.

Dosage

Extract: 120 to 240 milligrams daily, in 3 doses. Plan to take it for at least eight weeks before improvement shows.

Capsules: Depending on capsule strength of the product you buy, use the same amount as the above recommended dosage. The standard dose is 40 to 60 milligrams. Buy a quality product and read the label. Look for products marked "24/6," an indication the product contains 24 percent flavone glycosides and 6 percent terpenes.

GINSENG (*Panax ginseng*—Chinese/Korean/Japanese; *Panax quinquefolius*—American)

Common names: Man root, life root, heal-all 'seng
Medicinal part: Root
Description: Chinese ginseng is different from the American variety, but both have a fleshy, multibranched root. Due to its popularity, world trade in ginseng comes exclusively from cultivated plants; few are left remaining in the wild.

Called "the king of herbs" in the Orient, ginseng stimulates the entire body to overcome stress, fatigue, and weakness. Used in China for over 5000 years, ginseng was used by Arab physicians as early as the 9th century C.E. Marco Polo encountered the herb in

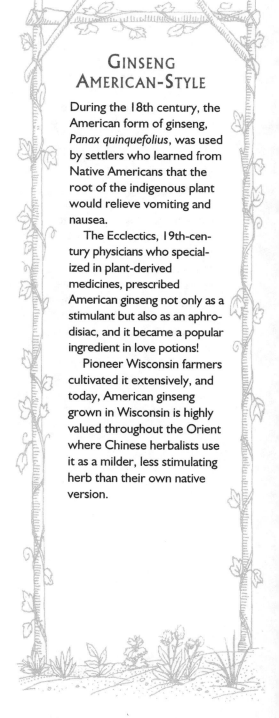

GINSENG AMERICAN-STYLE

During the 18th century, the American form of ginseng, *Panax quinquefolius*, was used by settlers who learned from Native Americans that the root of the indigenous plant would relieve vomiting and nausea.

The Ecclectics, 19th-century physicians who specialized in plant-derived medicines, prescribed American ginseng not only as a stimulant but also as an aphrodisiac, and it became a popular ingredient in love potions!

Pioneer Wisconsin farmers cultivated it extensively, and today, American ginseng grown in Wisconsin is highly valued throughout the Orient where Chinese herbalists use it as a milder, less stimulating herb than their own native version.

GREEK HAY

Long before its seeds became a popular remedy for human ills, fenugreek was used to treat sick animals. One of the oldest medicinal herbs, ancient Egyptian women used it to ease childbirth and increase milk flow. As a tea, it is commonly used to soothe gastric upsets suffered by tourists. Recent Western research has shown it to have hypoglycemic properties. The oil was used to make a skin ointment. In India, fenugreek seeds are a traditional treatment for diabetes. A recent study showed that the seeds lowered serum cholesterol levels by 14 percent in 60 noninsulin-dependent diabetic patients.

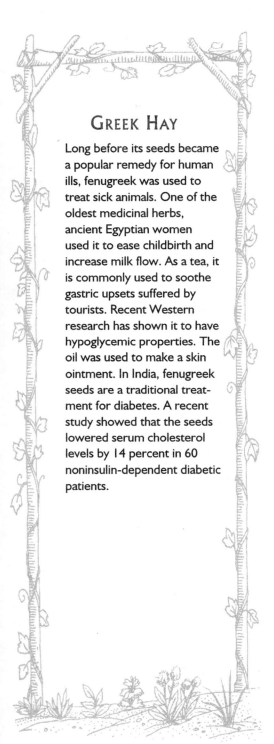

his travels and called it "the wonder of the world." King Louis XIV was visited by the king of Siam who presented him with a root, which the Sun King proceeded to have his gardeners cultivate. Ginseng quickly became popular with wealthy Europeans, who used it to combat exhaustion and debility—for which it is still used today. It is also suggested for fever, inflammations, respiratory illnesses, depression, immune system boosting, menstrual cramps, and to ease the labor of childbirth.

Ginseng

Probably more has been written and published about ginseng than any other herb, and since 1975, the volume has increased substantially. Still, hard scientific evidence of *how* the herb works or if, in fact, it does work is scarce. Though ginseng has been used for centuries in Asia as a "cure-all," investigators today are just beginning to understand this controversial herb's components and their effects or claimed results.

Varro E. Tyler, Ph.D., and consultant to *Prevention* magazine warns that quality is a problem due to the lack of standards. Consumers are advised to buy only standardized products with guaranteed potency from manufacturers with the highest reputations for ethics and standards. Red ginseng is considered to be of superior quality.

Dosage

Capsules: Follow the manufacturer's directions on the label. Milligram amounts can vary widely.

Infusion: Powdered ginseng can be used to make a tea; use 3 to 10 grams in 500 milliliters of water as a general tonic.

Caution: Do not exceed 5 to 10 grams daily and do not combine with vitamin C, which can prevent absorption.

GOLDENSEAL

"I am informed that the Cherokee cure it [cancer] with a plant which is thought to be the Hydrastis canadensis," wrote Benjamin Smith Barton in 1798. Today we call this plant goldenseal. A traditional healing herb of Native Americans, the

LADY'S MANTLE, LICORICE, AND LUNGWORT

Only a small number of herbs begin with the letter L, most of minor importance. Herb Mindell's *Herb Bible* contains references to lady's mantle, licorice, and lungwort.

Lady's mantle and other herbs with the word *lady* or *mother* as part of their names indicate gynecological uses. Lady's mantle was used specifically for heavy menstrual bleeding and vaginal itching as well as topically on wounds. During the 15th and 16th centuries it was popular on the battlefields of Europe. Arab women believe lady's mantle restores youth and beauty. It is commonly used as an infusion (1 tablespoon of dried herb to a cup of hot water) or sold commercially as an ointment for vaginal itching.

Licorice is a root that has been used for thousands of years to treat colds, coughs, ulcers, and infections. However, it has come under controversy due to recent scientific studies of its toxic side effects. What we know as licorice candy is actually flavored with anise oil, which is entirely safe.

True licorice candy is more readily available in Europe and England, where it is extremely popular. Licorice's principal component is glycyrrihizin, which accounts both for its sweetness and its danger. Recently, deglycyrrihizinated licorice products have appeared on the American market, but the pure substance is a potent botanical that must be used with caution.

Lungwort, as its name implies, is used to treat coughs, hoarseness, and mild lung problems. A 15th-century concept called the Doctrine of Signatures, espoused the belief that God shaped herbs in ways that showed their uses. Lungwort is an example of this notion, as its leaves are spotted in a manner similar to the appearance of actual lung tissue.

Also used to counteract diarrhea, lungwort is recommended for viral colds that are accompanied by stomach upset. It is usually taken daily as a tea made by steeping 1 tablespoon of the dry herb in a cup of hot water.

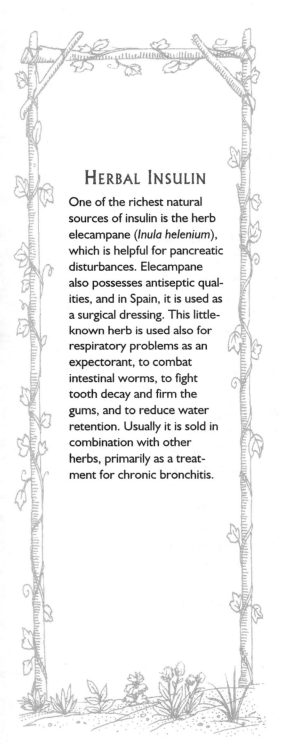

HERBAL INSULIN

One of the richest natural sources of insulin is the herb elecampane (*Inula helenium*), which is helpful for pancreatic disturbances. Elecampane also possesses antiseptic qualities, and in Spain, it is used as a surgical dressing. This little-known herb is used also for respiratory problems as an expectorant, to combat intestinal worms, to fight tooth decay and firm the gums, and to reduce water retention. Usually it is sold in combination with other herbs, primarily as a treatment for chronic bronchitis.

Cherokee used it for indigestion, local inflammations, and to improve the appetite. The Iroquois used it for whooping cough, liver problems, fevers, and heart disease. Introduced into Europe in 1760, this broad-spectrum herb was listed in the United States Pharmacopoeia until 1926. Considered one of the best general herbal remedies, it is becoming increasingly popular as a cleanser for mucous conditions, gastroenteritis, and vaginal discharge, and for digestive problems and PMS.

HAWTHORN (*Crataegus oxyacantha*)

Common names: May bush, May tree, thorn-apple, whitethorn

Medicinal parts: Berries (fruit), flowering tops

Description: A small deciduous tree with white bark and extremely hard wood, hawthorn, true to its name, has sharp thorns as well as aromatic white flowers and bright red fruits (which we consider berries). There are about 900 American species of hawthorn.

Hawthorn might well be called the "help for your heart herb," as it has been scientifically proven to lower high blood pressure, a prime risk factor for heart disease. It's also an excellent antioxidant that eliminates free radicals, the dangerous agents that roam the body and can cause damage to blood vessels, leading to atherosclerosis.

Hawthorn also contains rutin, a substance that reduces the formation of plaque, a build-up of which can block blood flow and possibly lead to stroke or a heart attack. Hawthorn is also effective against arrhythmia, a potentially dangerous heart rhythm disturbance. It can be used to improve strength and circulation in people with congestive heart failure.

If your family has a history of heart disease, you would be well advised to take hawthorn on a daily basis to strengthen your cardiac system before trouble develops. If you already have heart disease, ask your doctor about adding a daily dose of hawthorn to your medications. This herb has been shown to promote overall improvement in heart health and blood flow, ease angina and shortness of breath, and reduce swollen ankles.

"A WICKED WEED"

Although ancient Chinese, Greek, and Roman physicians all recommended hops as a digestive aid and treatment for stomach ailments, it was practically unknown in the West until about a thousand years ago, when brewers of English ale began using it as a preservative, which changed the taste of the brew. As the English take their ale seriously, this "additive" enraged the ale-drinking public, who complained to their King, Henry VIII, himself an ale traditionalist. Calling hops "a wicked weed that would endanger the people," King Henry banned the herb—which turned ale into beer—from use in brewing. His son and heir, Edward VI, who wasn't old enough to drink alcohol!—rescinded the ban in 1552, no doubt at the urging of his adult advisors, who recognized that the making of beer using hops as an ingredient turned a minor spring vegetable into a major cash crop.

Hops farmers soon began to notice that their pickers suffered two peculiar effects: They tired quickly when working, and the female pickers got their menstrual periods earlier than normal. As a result of their observations, hops became the herb of choice for sedation as well as an herb used by women to bring on their periods.

Science has since recognized the remarkable power of hops as a sedative. It has a calming effect on the body, soothes muscle spasms, relieves nervous tension, and promotes restful sleep. If you suffer from insomnia, make a tea with 1 teaspoon of dried hops in a cup of boiling water and drink at bedtime. Capsules are also available. Externally, an old-fashioned cure for sleeplessness is to sleep on a small pillowcase filled with hops sprinkled with alcohol.

HORSERADISH

Horseradish root possesses an antibiotic recommended for respiratory and urinary infections. It can be used internally to clear nasal passages and as a general cleanser for the entire body. It is available already grated in bottles at the supermarket. Look in the refrigerated section.

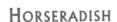

MOTHER'S MILK

Named for the milky white juice of its leaves, milk thistle's technical name, marianum, is the result of a legend. According to the legend, after being touched by a drop of milk from the breast of the Virgin Mary, the leaf veins turned milky white. This legend may account for the use of cooked milk thistle in the diets of European wet nurses, who believed it increased lactation.

Dosage

Tea: Use 1 tablespoon of dried berries to 1 cup of boiling water and steep for 10 minutes. Strain. Drink 1 cup daily.

Tablets: Take one 300-milligram tablet daily.

Tincture: Mix 1 tablespoon daily with any liquid.

MILK THISTLE (*Silybum marianum, Carduus marianus*)

Common names: Mary thistle, St. Mary's thistle, Our Lady's thistle

Medicinal parts: Leaves, fruit (seeds)

Description: Milk thistle is native to the Mediterranean and has been naturalized in California and the eastern United States. An annual or biennial, it grows up to 3 feet high and large, solitary, purple "thistles," or flower heads, appear from June to August.

Milk thistle, like dandelion, is often the gardener's bane, but herbalists and naturopathic physicians consider it a potent weapon against liver damage. Its use to support liver function goes back at least to the 1st century C.E. Like many herbal remedies, it got lost with the advent of pharmaceuticals, and as recently as 1947, the *U.S. Dispensatory* gave it short shrift—one paragraph about its history.

However, recent clinical research, especially by German scientists, indicate that milk thistle is indeed effective. Over three hundred studies conducted since the late 1960s report no toxic side effects. The "seeds," which are actually its fruit, contain a bioflavonoid complex that has powerful antioxidant abilities. According to Stephen Foster's *101 Medicinal Herbs*, standardized milk thistle seed preparations have been shown to change the cell structure of the outer liver membrane, thus preventing toxic chemicals from entering while stimulating the liver to generate new cells. Milk thistle may be of value against viral hepatitis as well.

German health authorities have endorsed the use of milk thistle as a supportive treatment for inflammatory liver conditions and cirrhosis, but it has value as a preventative as well because it stimulates protein synthesis, which results in an

FROM MEDICINE TO MARTINI

A Dutch pharmacist concocted a preparation with juniper berries, to be used as a diuretic, and called it ginever, from which we get the word *gin*. Gin became enormously popular with the English, who, when in India, mixed it with quinine to avoid malaria, creating gin-and-tonic. Juniper and its volatile oil—in which over 105 constituents have been found—have a tradition in folk medicine as a diuretic and for carminative action. Excessive use may cause kidney irritation, and as juniper is hazardous to pregnant women, it should be used cautiously with medical approval.

increase in the production of new liver cells to replace damaged old ones. Dr. Andrew Weil strongly recommends milk thistle for anyone who regularly consumes alcohol or is exposed to toxic chemicals.

The liver is our second largest organ and is essential to overall health. It is also the only organ in the body with the ability to rejuvenate itself. It is the main source of detoxification, especially from alcohol, nicotine (including second-hand smoke), and carbon monoxide. As humans are daily exposed to more and more pollutants, our livers are being required to work overtime to expel these toxins. Therefore, almost everyone can benefit by supplementing their diets with this lowly weed.

Dosage

Capsules: The primary form in which milk thistle is marketed in the United States is in capsule form. Capsules containing 200 milligrams of a concentrated extract, which represents 140 milligrams of silymarin. One to three tablets a day are recommended; or, follow instructions on the manufacturer's label.

PARSLEY

Parsley is a natural antispasmodic that relieves gas as well as a natural diuretic. Its expectorant properties make it useful for coughs and asthma. Studies are underway to determine if parsley contains a substance that prevents cancer cells from multiplying. Parsley helps the anemic person by increasing iron content in the blood. The herb is a good nutrient, but the volatile oil from the seeds can be toxic. Pregnant women should not ingest parsley juice or oil. Chop parsley leaves and use raw as a salad ingredient or add them to cooked foods, such as bulgur wheat, rice, or stew. To make a tea, steep leaves and stems in hot water. Chewing a spring of parsley after a meal freshens the breath and eliminates "garlic breath."

Medicinally, parsley is controversial. Tyler's *New Honest Herbal* dismisses it as "essentially worthless." However, the German authority Rudolph Fritz Weiss, M.D., in a medical text called *Herbal Medicine*, says it is "a major medicinal plant."

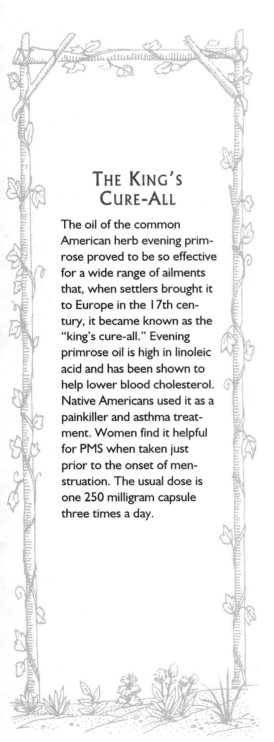

THE KING'S CURE-ALL

The oil of the common American herb evening primrose proved to be so effective for a wide range of ailments that, when settlers brought it to Europe in the 17th century, it became known as the "king's cure-all." Evening primrose oil is high in linoleic acid and has been shown to help lower blood cholesterol. Native Americans used it as a painkiller and asthma treatment. Women find it helpful for PMS when taken just prior to the onset of menstruation. The usual dose is one 250 milligram capsule three times a day.

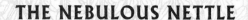

THE NEBULOUS NETTLE

About the only thing everyone agrees on about the nettle plant is that it stings. Says Varro E. Tyler in *The Honest Herbal*:

> *One would think that a high-technology society capable of splitting the atom and sending a man to the moon would long ago have learned everything there is to know about the stinging nettle. Not so. Even the agent responsible for the skin irritation produced by contact with the leaves of this common plant remains nearly as much a mystery to twentieth-century scientists as it did to the first caveman who stumbled against it.*

Traditionally a folk remedy for hay fever and other allergies, the entire plant is collected before it flowers and dried to make capsules or tea. Some herbalists claim it is good for vaginal infections such as candida and that its use will reduce excess menstrual flow. Animal studies have suggested nettle can lower blood sugar, a finding that might be of use to diabetics in the future.

In Germany, health authorities have approved extract of nettle root for the treatment of urinary retention brought on by benign enlargement of the prostate gland. However, studies have not verified nettle's traditional use. It can be taken as a commercially produced capsule for hay fever, or used to make a tea for hemorrhoids. Take your pick, but *pick carefully* if harvesting the fresh plant. Its fierce sting has given us the word *nettlesome* for anything that irritates us beyond our toleration.

Rich in chlorophyll, young shoots contain about the same amount of vitamins A and C as spinach—but *never* eat nettles raw.

St. Hildegard of Bingen, the famous medieval German herbalist, believed that a wine made from parsley improved blood circulation and helped heart conditions. Her recipe for making parsley wine is as follows:

Combine a dozen or so large sprigs of fresh washed parsley with 1 quart of red or white wine and 2 teaspoons of white-wine vinegar. Boil the mixture for 10 minutes. Add 9 ounces of honey and mix well. Strain the cooled mixture and pour into sterilized bottles. Take 1 teaspoon three times a day. It can be diluted with water for a beverage.

PEPPERMINT (*Mentha x piperita*)

Common name: Mint (sometimes erroneously called spearmint)

Medicinal part: Leaves, harvested before the plant flowers

Description: Peppermint is a natural hybrid that was found sprouting in a field of spearmint in England in 1696. Ever since, it has been intensively cultivated for its fragrant volatile oil. It does not breed from seed, is vegetatively propagated, and comes in numerous cultivated varieties.

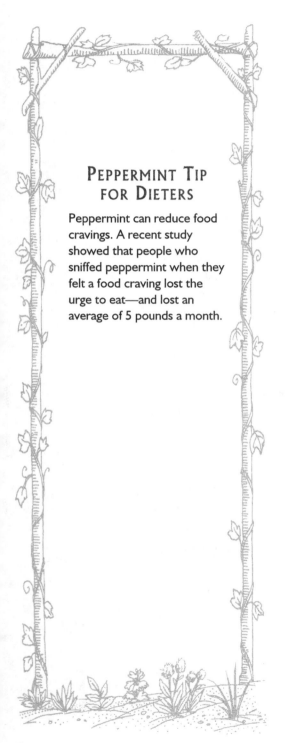

Peppermint

An extremely common herb, peppermint is known for its stimulating and carminative properties and is used to treat indigestion and flatulence. It is also used for infant colic. Studies show that peppermint acts by stimulating the gastric lining, thus lessening the amount of time food spends in the stomach. It also acts as a relaxant on the stomach muscles and induces burping, which alleviates the unpleasant feeling of fullness.

Until the 17th century, all mints, of which there are at least thirty species, were used in much the same way. However, peppermint, designated as *M. piperita*, is the preferred mint variety for medicinal use in the West.

Its use includes easing heartburn, stomachache, nausea, and vomiting. The nauseous type of migraine headaches are often helped by peppermint, which has a calming effect overall.

PEPPERMINT TIP FOR DIETERS

Peppermint can reduce food cravings. A recent study showed that people who sniffed peppermint when they felt a food craving lost the urge to eat—and lost an average of 5 pounds a month.

Peppermint is generally considered safe, but the FDA has banned the nonprescriptive sale of the oil as a digestive aid. In Germany, however, health authorities have declared both peppermint and its volatile oil to be effective spasmolytics, antibacterial agents, and promoters of gastric secretions.

In his book, *Herb Bible*, Earl Mindell says that it is an excellent substitute for coffee and tea and that "it works better than aspirin or acetaminophen [against headache]." He suggests combining a cup of strong peppermint tea with a 15-minute rest and elaborates that "considering all the things that peppermint can do, no home medicine cabinet should be without it!"

Do not confuse peppermint with spearmint. They are quite different, although similar in appearance. Peppermint's therapeutic quality is due to menthol, a substance not present in spearmint, which is used only as a flavoring agent.

Peppermint teas come in any number of commercially prepared mixtures. Read the label before buying to make sure you are getting real peppermint and not just a mint-flavored tea.

Dosage

Tea: The most common form is an infusion of 1 tablespoon, or one commercial tea bag, with 8 ounces of boiling water. Steep 5 minutes or more and drink as needed.

Caution: Do not give peppermint tea to infants without the approval of your pediatrician.

RASPBERRY (*Rubus strigosus*: North America)
Common name: Wild red raspberry
Medicinal parts: Leaves, fruit
Description: Wild red raspberry is a shrubby plant that is indigenous to the untended fields and forests of North America. A durable root produces the prickly stem with alternating, feather-like leaves. During the plant's second year, white cup-shaped flowers appear in the spring and summer. The red fruit is edible, and ripens during the summer.

Dosage: Steep 1 oz. leaves in 2 cups water for 15 minutes. Take 2 cups a day.

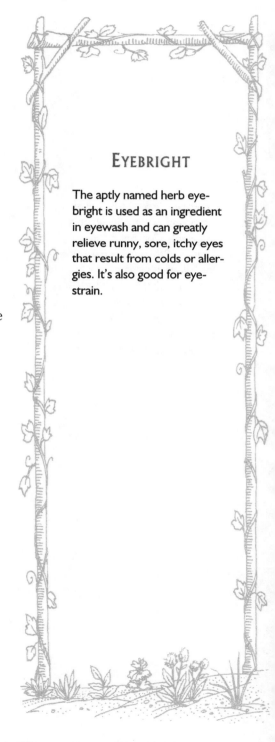

EYEBRIGHT

The aptly named herb eyebright is used as an ingredient in eyewash and can greatly relieve runny, sore, itchy eyes that result from colds or allergies. It's also good for eyestrain.

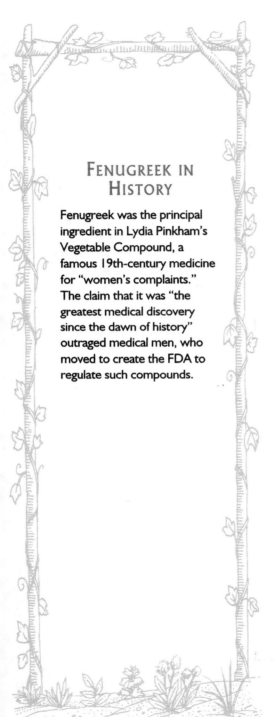

FENUGREEK IN
HISTORY

Fenugreek was the principal
ingredient in Lydia Pinkham's
Vegetable Compound, a
famous 19th-century medicine
for "women's complaints."
The claim that it was "the
greatest medical discovery
since the dawn of history"
outraged medical men, who
moved to create the FDA to
regulate such compounds.

Raspberry Leaves are harvested from the red raspberry bush
(which is different from the black raspberry); the bush grows
abundantly and easily, to the point of becoming invasive.

In the days when midwives were pregnant women's primary
health care providers, and "natural" childbirth was not an option
but a necessity, raspberry leaves were the midwives' herb of
choice for their patients, who were advised to drink it daily
during the last three months of pregnancy (but not early on) in
order to promote an easy delivery by tonifying the uterus.

After the child was born, new mothers were to take raspberry tea for several weeks to aid the uterus's return to a
normal state. It was also used in nonpregnant women to ease
menstrual cramps. It has astringent and antispasmodic properties, which are especially applicable to the womb.

Other uses for raspberry leaves are as an infusion to make
a mouthwash for sore gums, sore throats, and mouth ulcers. Dr.
Shealy, in his *Illustrated Encyclopedia of Natural Remedies*, says
that it can be used for children's diarrhea and oral thrush by
putting raspberry leaf tea into a sterilized spray bottle and
spraying into the mouth of the infant three or four times a day.
He further recommends using standardized forms of the leaves
and following the dose instructions on the packet.

ROSEMARY (*Rosmarinus officinalis*: Mediterranean)
Common name: Rosemary
Medicinal part: Leaves, flowering tops
Description: Rosemary is an evergreen shrub whose origins can be traced to the Mediterranean area. Today,
Rosemary is widely cultivated for its aromatic leaves
and as a kitchen seasoning. The pale blue (sometimes white) flowers bloom during April
and May, or later in cooler climates.

Rosemary leaves have a long traditional
history. They grow on a late-flowering
woody shrub, which is abundant in the
Mediterranean area. Crushing a few
leaves between the fingers releases a pungent aromatic scent. The old saying,

Rosemary

"Rosemary is for remembrance," may have some truth in it; according to Dr. Shealy, rosemary enhances the memory by improving the circulation.

Dosage:

Infusion: Steep 1 teaspoon dried flowering tops or leaves in ¹/₂ cup water. Take up to 1 cup a day.

Tincture: A dose is from 5 to 20 drops.

It is said to lift the spirits and is used to improve circulation, as a carminative, as a bitter but gentle tonic, as a gargle for sore throats, and to relieve depression and headaches associated with gastric upsets. Large doses should be avoided by pregnant women unless they are under the care of a qualified herbalist. It should not be used to treat headaches and migraines that feel "hot," advises Dr. Shealy. Otherwise, he says, standard doses may be used freely. He also states that 15 drops of the essential oil added to a bath will ease muscular tension, improve circulation, and lift the spirits. Rosemary has also been widely used as a preservative for food. And Dr. Shealy suggests rosemary vinegar as a treatment for dandruff.

SAGE LEAVES *(Salvia officinalis)*

Common name: Garden sage

Medicinal part: Leaves

Description: Sage is a shrubby perennial plant that can be found growing wild along the shorelines of Mediterranean and southern European countries. It is cultivated worldwide as a strong kitchen spice. Purple, blue, or white two-lipped flowers growing in whorls can be found blooming in June and July.

Sage leaves are a common garden and culinary herb. The genus name, *Salvia*, suggests health, and sage was traditionally thought to promote long life and, consequently, wisdom; hence a *sage* is a wise person.

Sage has astringent, stimulant, antiseptic, carminative, antispasmodic, and nervine properties. It is generally strengthening and a good tonic for women. It was considered a general tonic for the blood throughout Europe and America.

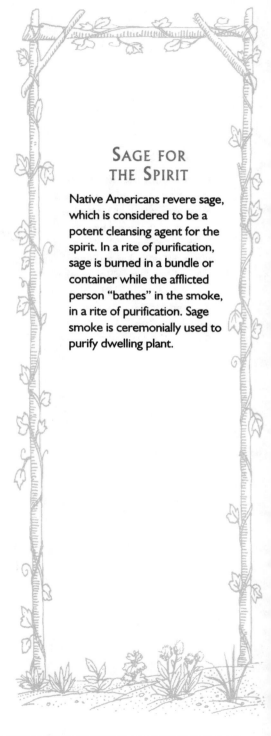

SAGE FOR THE SPIRIT

Native Americans revere sage, which is considered to be a potent cleansing agent for the spirit. In a rite of purification, sage is burned in a bundle or container while the afflicted person "bathes" in the smoke, in a rite of purification. Sage smoke is ceremonially used to purify dwelling plant.

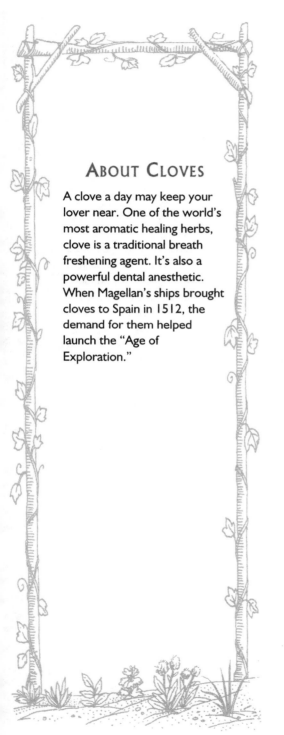

ABOUT CLOVES

A clove a day may keep your lover near. One of the world's most aromatic healing herbs, clove is a traditional breath freshening agent. It's also a powerful dental anesthetic. When Magellan's ships brought cloves to Spain in 1512, the demand for them helped launch the "Age of Exploration."

Its uses are for depression and nervous exhaustion, post-viral fatigue, and general debility. Dr. Shealy lists it as an antidote to anxiety and confusion in the elderly, as well as for indigestion, flatulence, loss of appetite, night sweating, chronic or recurrent coughs, and as a gargle and mouthwash for sore throats, laryngitis, tonsillitis, mouth ulcers, and inflamed gums.

Its antiseptic properties make it good as a wash for wounds; it can be made into a poultice with cider vinegar.

Herbalist Susun S. Weed from Woodstock, New York, author of *Wise Woman Ways: Menopausal Years*, says that just 1 cup of sage tea can stave off "hot flashes," or excessive sweating, for up to two days. To make a tea, she suggests adding 4 heaping tablespoons of dried sage to a cup of hot water, covering the container tightly, and allowing the brew to steep for four hours before straining and drinking. She cautions women not to drink more than 1 cup per day due to the possible side effects of thujone in sage.

Sage

Sage is to be avoided by anyone allergic to aspirin (salicylates), and medicinal doses should not be taken by pregnant or nursing women, nor for those with epilepsy. Most authorities agree sage should be used moderately. Penelope Ody, in *The Complete Medicinal Herbal*, warns that excess use can produce symptoms of poisoning, and Dr. Tyler warns against the agent thujone found in sage.

For safety's sake, when using as a medicinal, always use standard doses and follow the instructions for use on the label. The small amounts used in cooking are quite safe as heat apparently destroys the volatile thujone.

Dosage:
Infusion: Steep 1 teaspoon leaves in ½ cup water for 30 minutes. Take 1 cup daily, a tablespoonful at a time.
Powder: Take ¼ to ½ teaspoon powdered leaves at a time.
Tincture: Take 15 to 40 drops, 3 or 4 times a day.

SAW PALMETTO (*Serenoa serrulata*)

Common name: Saw palmetto

Medicinal part: Berries

Description: Saw Palmetto is the fruit of a small palm-like plant found in the West Indies and the United States. Its berries are dried after gathering during fall and winter. It is plentiful along the southeastern coast of Florida and the Gulf Coast. Indians native to these areas recognized the medicinal qualities of saw palmetto, and in the 1870s it began to be recognized within the contemporary medical community, being added to the *United States Pharmacopoeia* in 1905.

Native Americans used saw palmetto roots to treat snakebite, kidney problems, high blood pressure, and neuralgia. Today, research has renewed interest in the saw palmetto, which is claimed to be effective as a treatment for prostate enlargement and cystitis. Tests on patients with this condition, called BPH (nonmalignant enlargement of the prostate gland), have been extensive but controversial. French and German doctors regularly use saw palmetto as a treatment for enlarged prostate and related symptoms, but there can be side effects. All authorities agree that no one with this condition should self-medicate but should rely on professional health care providers for diagnosis and advice about treatment. In addition, pregnant women, especially in the early terms, should not use the herb without consulting their doctors.

Dosage:

Infusion: Use ¹/₂ teaspoon crushed berries to 1 cup hot water. Take 1 to 2 cups daily.

Tincture: Use 20 to 30 drops, and take 3 times daily.

ST. JOHN'S WORT (*Hypericum perforatum*)

Common names: Amber, goatweed, johnswort, Klamath weed, Tipton weed

Medicinal part: The herb

Description: St. John's wort is a shrubby perennial plant commonly found in dry, gravelly soils, fields, and sunny places in many

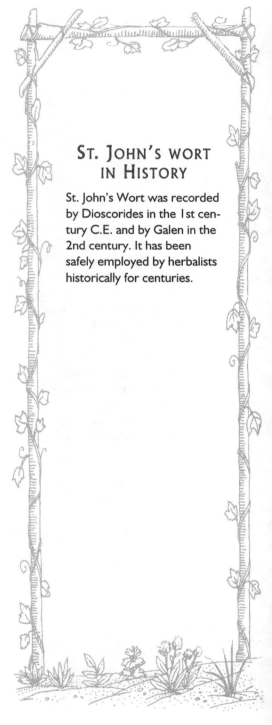

ST. JOHN'S WORT IN HISTORY

St. John's Wort was recorded by Dioscorides in the 1st century C.E. and by Galen in the 2nd century. It has been safely employed by herbalists historically for centuries.

parts of the world, including eastern North America and the Pacific coast. A woody, branched root produces many round stems which put out runners from the base. Yellow flowers, whose petals are dotted with black along the margins, appear from June to September. The fruit is a three-celled capsule containing small, dark brown seeds. The whole plant has a turpentine-like odor.

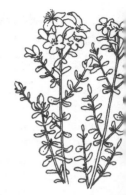

St. John's Wort

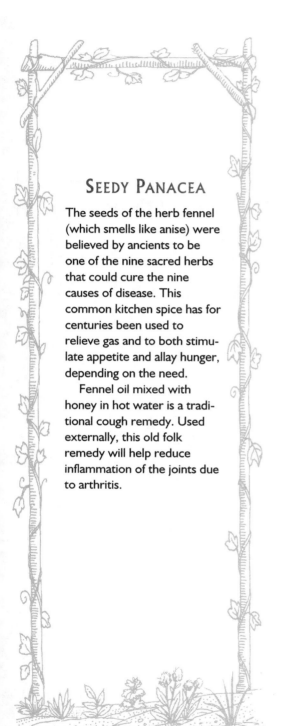

SEEDY PANACEA

The seeds of the herb fennel (which smells like anise) were believed by ancients to be one of the nine sacred herbs that could cure the nine causes of disease. This common kitchen spice has for centuries been used to relieve gas and to both stimulate appetite and allay hunger, depending on the need.

Fennel oil mixed with honey in hot water is a traditional cough remedy. Used externally, this old folk remedy will help reduce inflammation of the joints due to arthritis.

St. John's wort, popular in Europe for years, received an enormous amount of media attention when, in June of 1997, millions of Americans saw a segment on the ABC television show *20/20* that reported positively on the herb's ability to treat depression. After this episode was aired, millions of Americans rushed to their health stores to purchase St. John's wort, the sales of which rose to dramatic proportions.

Depression—whether mild or severe—is one of the most prevalent conditions from which Americans suffer, and many of them never seek medical or professional treatment for the problem. Self-diagnosis is prevalent and, therefore, so is self-treatment. Due to the sheer complexity of the human psyche and the multitude of factors that can influence the body and the interaction between the two, depression is not a single-issue ailment—nor are herbs made of a single component. Medical studies of St. John's wort generally show it to be positive, and its therapeutic use for mood disorders, anxiety, and the like is approved by German health authorities.

No one seems to know just what it is about St. John's wort that improves depressive states. Since herbs in their pure form have many constituents that make up the chemical components that give each its own individual personality, it is entirely possible that St. John's wort functions through a variety of its components.

Even before it attracted widespread media coverage in the United States, it was widely distributed in Europe, Asia, and northern Africa. *Better Nutrition* published an article in February 1996 saying that "St. John's wort [is] effective medicine for depression, infection, and more," and that the herb, called *Hypericum perforatum* in Latin, already outsells Prozac twenty to one in Germany, and it is available at about ¹/₄ the cost of the 10-year-old antidepressant drug sold by Eli Lilly that has become one of the world's top-selling pharmaceuticals.

According to Michael T. Murray, N.D., author of *Natural Alternatives to Prozac,* about 25 supervised, double-blind studies involving a total of 1,592 patients who received positive effects from St. John's wort reported that it improved psychological problems like depression, anxiety, and sleep disorders without side effects.

It should be noted that fair-skinned people especially should avoid exposure to sunlight when taking St. John's wort and that the herb should not be combined with Prozac. In his book *Herbs for Your Health*, herbalist Stephen Foster warns that the two may interact dangerously. Murray also makes the point that drugs like Prozac may only *mask* the underlying causes of depression and he suggests that St. John's wort should be used as a safer, nonaddictive antidepressant aid until the true causes of the depression are uncovered and treated properly.

Since the emotional and physical needs of humans are so closely interwoven, and since plants are capable of acting on the human emotional as well as physical systems, herbs may be much preferable as treatments than synthesized drugs. But no one ever should treat depression lightly, and neither St. John's wort nor other herbal treatments should be used to replace prescription drugs being taken by people who have been diagnosed with clinical depression.

Occasional use of St. John's wort (while avoiding sun) can be considered a safe treatment for "the blues" that most everyone is subject to feeling. Dr. Shealy points out that St. John's wort in a standard dose may take a week to show a lift in the depression; however, many antidepressant prescription drugs can take a month or more to show results.

In addition to its popular use to alleviate mood disorders, St. John's wort is popular in Europe as a remedy for gastrointestinal disorders. Externally, it is used as an antiseptic and analgesic for wounds, rashes, shingles, cold sores, and herpes. Ointments prepared from the herb are said to help sciatic and back pain.

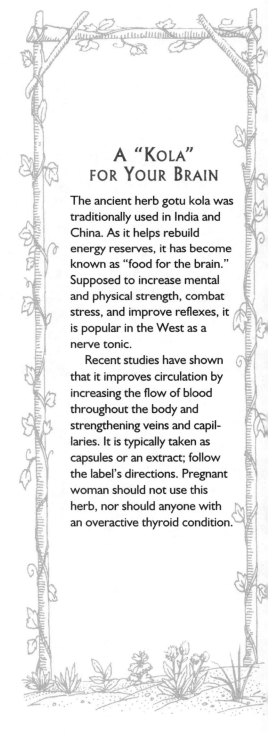

A "KOLA" FOR YOUR BRAIN

The ancient herb gotu kola was traditionally used in India and China. As it helps rebuild energy reserves, it has become known as "food for the brain." Supposed to increase mental and physical strength, combat stress, and improve reflexes, it is popular in the West as a nerve tonic.

Recent studies have shown that it improves circulation by increasing the flow of blood throughout the body and strengthening veins and capillaries. It is typically taken as capsules or an extract; follow the label's directions. Pregnant woman should not use this herb, nor should anyone with an overactive thyroid condition.

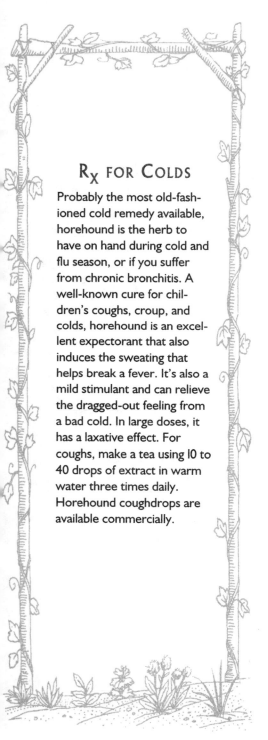

Rx FOR COLDS

Probably the most old-fashioned cold remedy available,
horehound is the herb to
have on hand during cold and
flu season, or if you suffer
from chronic bronchitis. A
well-known cure for chil-
dren's coughs, croup, and
colds, horehound is an excellent expectorant that also
induces the sweating that
helps break a fever. It's also a
mild stimulant and can relieve
the dragged-out feeling from
a bad cold. In large doses, it
has a laxative effect. For
coughs, make a tea using 10 to
40 drops of extract in warm
water three times daily.
Horehound coughdrops are
available commercially.

Dosage:

Infusion: Steep 1 teaspoon dried herb in $\frac{1}{2}$ cup water for 5 minutes, covered. Take warm, $\frac{1}{2}$ cup before breakfast and $\frac{1}{2}$ cup when going to bed.

Oil extract: Take 10 to 15 drops in water. To make, put fresh flowers and leaves in a jar and fill with olive oil. Close the jar and leave it in a sunny or warm place for 6 to 7 weeks, shaking it often. The oil will turn red. Strain the oil through a cloth. If a water layer appears when the oil has stood a while, decant or siphon it off. In a dark container, the oil will keep for up to 2 years.

This selective listing of herbs by no means covers the vast territory of herbs and their uses. There are literally hundreds of herbs (and plants) with medicinal uses. Some of these have been popular for centuries and are now being debunked. Others are simply ignored by everyone except dedicated herbalists. Still others have been studied extensively with inconclusive results. A few have been proved by modern science to do what both ancient and modern herbalists have contended they can do.

For some herbalists, their profession is more like a calling than a vocation, and they can be most insistent about their beliefs. Others choose to accept historical and traditional uses of herbs as proof of their validity and have researched the vast litera-ture available on herbs and their properties. Still others, more sci-entific minded, require that herbs they recommend have effects that are attested to by current government-supported research, most of which has been done in Germany. Little research has been done in the United States because plant remedies cannot be patented, and, therefore, the profit incentive is missing.

As a result, while many European and British physicians routinely prescribe herbal medicines in addition to or instead of pharmaceuticals, most American physicians remain either igno-rant of herbal remedies or hostile to them. If you are interested in having a doctor's opinion on any herbal remedies you would like to investigate or to take, there is a book now available, by Volker Schultz, Rudolf Hansel, and Varro E. Tyler, Ph.D., Sc.D., that was written especially for physicians called *Rational Phytotherapy: A Physicians' Guide to Herbal Medicine.*

Unfortunately, American medical schools ignore the history of healing, so many physicians aren't aware of the fact that many modern drugs are plant-based. For example, aspirin was originally created from white willow bark and meadowsweet; meadowsweet's Latin name *Spirea* provided the *spirin* in *aspirin*.

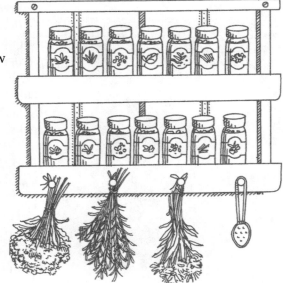

The situation is improving. Since 1986, the natural products branch of the National Cancer Institute has tested forty thousand plant samples—gathered from all over the world—in its search for treatments for AIDS and cancer. Yet, many doctors don't even know that approximately half of the drugs sold today in the United States are plant-derived, such as digitalis (from foxglove) and taxol (from the Pacific yew tree).

Some companies are willing to fund research and testing in hopes of winning profit-making patents for new products. But due to the difficulty of actually patenting plant substances used since antiquity as medicinals, most pharmaceutical firms have little incentive to invest money in extensive and expensive testing, which is needed to satisfy the FDA.

The situation is confusing also because botanicals are classified as "dietary supplements," not as drugs, even though many consumers use them medicinally. Thus, many herbal specialists think that the only way for herbal remedies to be scientifically tested for safety and that the only way to standardize industry practices to achieve greater consistency in product quality is for the government to become involved.

Despite uncertainties, and some specific warnings and restrictions given regarding certain herbals, especially for use by pregnant women, or in combination with other herbs or with prescription drugs, the general consensus is that side effects of herbal preparations are much less than those of pharmaceuticals, when taken as recommended.

An article in the May 1999 issue of the *AARP Bulletin* suggests that anyone wanting to take herbs do so with proper precaution.

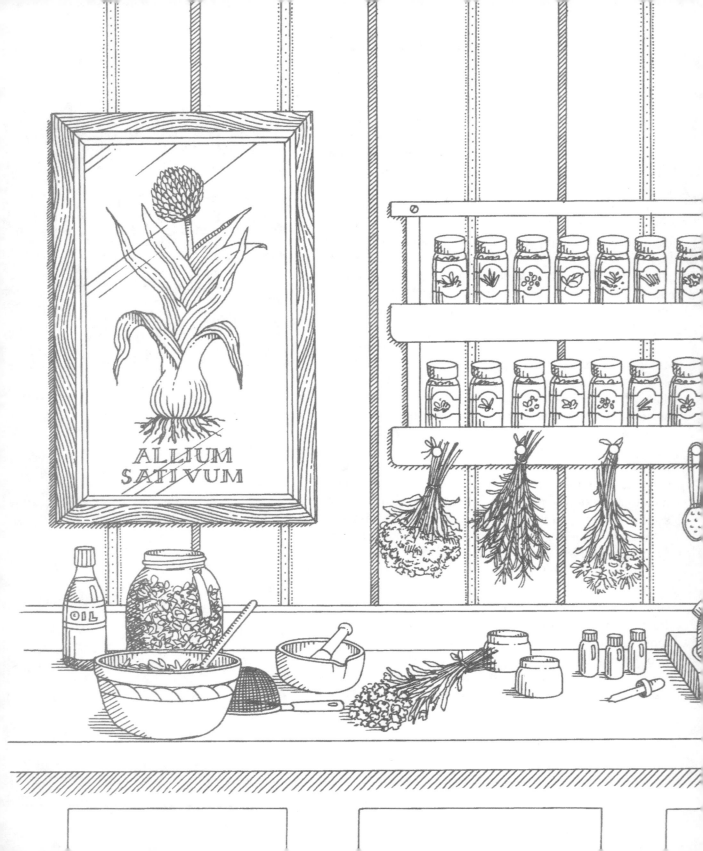

ALLIUM
SATIVUM

OIL

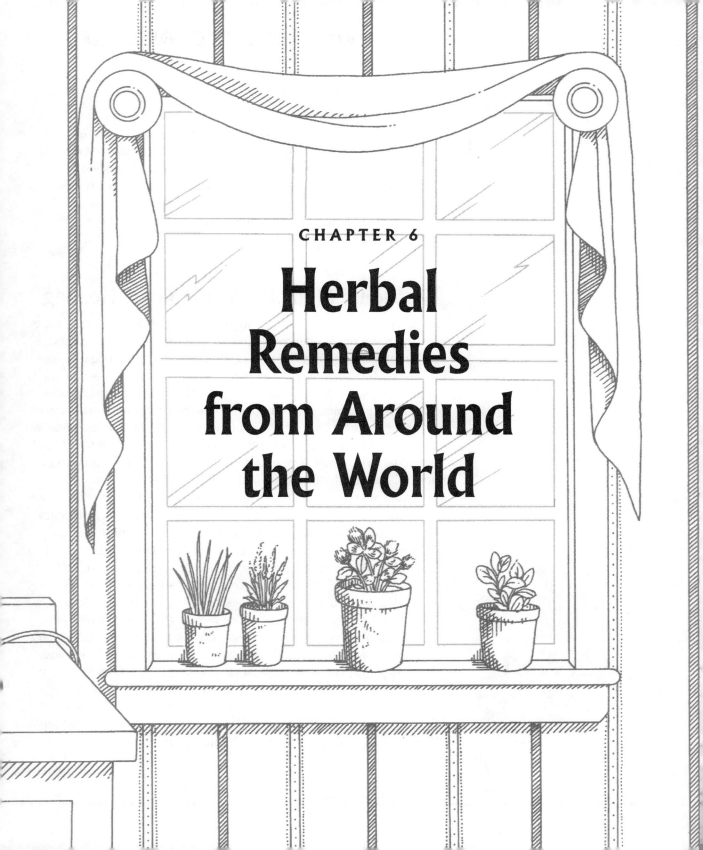

CHAPTER 6

Herbal Remedies from Around the World

Western scientific medicine is largely concerned with objective, nonpersonal, physiochemical explanations of disease as well as its technical control. In contrast, many traditional systems of healing are centered on the phenomenon of illness, namely, the personal and social experience of disease . . . . Where Western scientific medicine focuses on curing the disease, traditional medicine aims primarily at healing the illness—that is, managing the individual and social response to disease.

—David S. Sobel

Traditional Medicine and Holistic Healing

Our understanding of our own bodies began to emerge from the mists of shamanistic ritual, often reviled as superstition, about 5000 years ago. At that time, medical professionals and researchers began to seriously study the body and its functions in China, India, Greece, and Egypt. Although these early cultures had differences in language and religious philosophies, they approached the body from the same basic worldview, seeing it as a whole, a unity. In this worldview, the body is considered a unified system in which physical, mental, emotional, and spiritual factors operate together, not separately. Moreover, individual human life is considered to be at one with the universe itself.

Classical man saw sickness as the effect of a divine action, which could be cured only by another divine action; the divine sickness was to be cast out by a divine remedy. In *Incubation and Modern Psychotherapy*, C. A. Meier says, "The *divina afflictio* then contains its own diagnosis, therapy and prognosis, provided of course that the right attitude toward it is adopted."

At the classical sanctuaries of healing in ancient Greece, a distinctly spiritual atmosphere was created. Dedicated to the god of healing, these ancient "hospitals" had as their primary aim the connecting of the patient with his or her innermost depths, from where the healing would come. Removed from the distractions and disturbances of the outside world, patients were presented with the opportunity to themselves effect their cure, the elements of which already resided within them. When sickness is vested with such dignity, it has the inestimable advantage of being the agent of its own cure. Thus, what might be called spiritual homeopathy was practiced in the clinics of antiquity, through the medium of dreams and what today we call altered states of consciousness.

At the healing temples of Asklepios, both patient and doctor made ritual sacrifices, after which the patient retired into seclusion within the temple to await a dream message from a particular god about his or her illness and its cure. The mystery of recovery was a private matter between the individual and the god responsible for it. In principle, the physician was excluded from the process. Unfortunately, today modern medicine emphasizes using drugs and surgery to overcome disease rather than focusing solely on encouraging the body's own healing powers as the ancients did.

In our society, the correspondences between religion, magic, and medicine have been all but lost. Many members of the medical establishment have narrowed and restricted their view to the physical body and the material aspects of illness, health, and life itself. They do not—or will not—believe that nonphysical forces are what animate and support the manifest world, including that of the physical body.

The contributions of science to our health are important and valuable, but the mindset of the medical community too often does not allow for the interplay of all the energies of mind, body, and spirit. We ourselves must be responsible for recognizing our need for wholeness and integrating it into our lives. The necessity for healing—not only of ourselves but also of our societies and our planet—is immediate, even *urgent*. We should not wait for those who do not embrace the concept of wholeness exemplified in the use of herbs as medicine, a practice that goes around the world, to give us permission to explore our own natures—including body, mind, and spirit—and use them fully to heal ourselves and maintain health. With all the information now at our disposal, we have both the opportunity and the responsibility to empower ourselves with the wisdom of our ancestors and learn from their age-old methods of herbal usage.

According to tradition, Chinese wholeness is made up of two parts, yin, which represents the feminine principle, and *yang*, which is symbolic of the masculine principle. Together, yin and yang

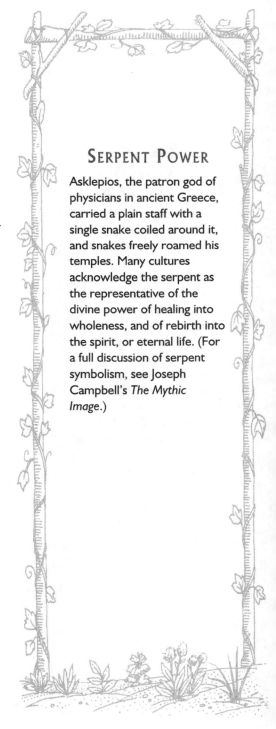

SERPENT POWER

Asklepios, the patron god of physicians in ancient Greece, carried a plain staff with a single snake coiled around it, and snakes freely roamed his temples. Many cultures acknowledge the serpent as the representative of the divine power of healing into wholeness, and of rebirth into the spirit, or eternal life. (For a full discussion of serpent symbolism, see Joseph Campbell's *The Mythic Image*.)

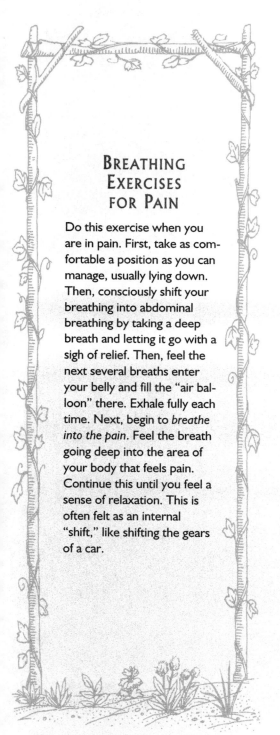

BREATHING EXERCISES FOR PAIN

Do this exercise when you are in pain. First, take as comfortable a position as you can manage, usually lying down. Then, consciously shift your breathing into abdominal breathing by taking a deep breath and letting it go with a sigh of relief. Then, feel the next several breaths enter your belly and fill the "air balloon" there. Exhale fully each time. Next, begin to *breathe into the pain*. Feel the breath going deep into the area of your body that feels pain. Continue this until you feel a sense of relaxation. This is often felt as an internal "shift," like shifting the gears of a car.

manifest the entire material universe and are naturally in perfect balance. They act like poles of a magnet, attracting each other, which produces movement and energy, or the life force, which is called *chi* or *qi*. Illness is a disruption of the balance of yin and yang and is corrected through rebalancing these two energies.

This idea of a universal life force includes the idea that the body possesses its own inner wisdom and healing powers. Already they are at work within you—repairing and replacing your cells, eliminating waste, nourishing tissues, fighting off germs, calming nerves, protecting you from infection, balancing your hormones, and, when necessary, healing contusions and wounds. Most of the time you are almost completely unaware of all this activity going on, but you can accelerate your body's healing power by learning to use it consciously.

Your body's healing power is as much a part of you as your ability to think, to feel, to make decisions, to make love, to live. It's always there, on duty and on guard around the clock. You can think of it as an entire army, headed by a commanding general who supervises its operations, immensely complicated as they are (no mere battlefield commander could possibly direct its functions). Each of your cells is a scientific genius, endowed with the ability to repair itself, as well as the capacity to renew and regenerate itself; in fact, every cell in your body replaces itself with a completely new cell every seven years. You literally produce a new body. Today, medical researchers are proving in the scientific laboratory what metaphysicans have known all along: When things get seriously out of balance through stress or trauma, balancing opposite tendencies can release inner healing powers.

The life force is a powerful one. Just think of the fact that a tiny blade of grass, pushing up from a speck of a seed in the soil below, can crack open a cement sidewalk. The question arises, If we have such amazing restorative powers, why do we get sick? There can be no completely definitive answer to that question, but a large part of the reason is that we suffer from self-inflicted conditions, most often derived from negative and traumatic emotional experiences that in turn afflict us with ongoing negative thought patterns, which often turn into illnesses.

THE HEALING POWER OF BREATH

Breath is life. When breath stops, life stops. The vital force of life comes into our bodies with our breath. Yet, we are mostly unaware of this and often neglect to breathe fully and deeply. Breath is the gateway to improved health and to amplified healing. Something we take for granted—for we could hardly function if we had to consciously remember to breathe—most of us are rarely aware of our breathing until it becomes impaired, by a cold or by shortness of breath. When we become aware of our breathing, we connect to the implicit order or realm of subtle energies within us. Breath is the link we have with our unconscious selves; it is the carrier not only of oxygen but also of information about our inner states. Awareness and control of breath allows us to consciously open ourselves to our innate healing powers.

Controlled breathing permits us to extract new energy from the air. Our physical bodies can store this energy in the same way food is stored as fat. When this subtle energy is in short supply, you feel down, listless, tired, and can get sick. When it is in abundant supply, you feel "up," energized, optimistic, and full of energy. Though the energy is subtle, it is very real.

Unfortunately, most adults are shallow breathers. They sip the air the way a Victorian lady sipped her cup of tea, and for the same reason—not to appear coarse. Taking in generous amounts of air seems impolite to many people, especially those who feel socially restricted and insecure about how others will view them. A good belly breath, like a good belly laugh, seems not to belong in polite company.

Breath, like food, nourishes our every cell and cleanses our blood. But, like anorexics, we insist on starving ourselves of this vital nutrient. The good news is that changing breathing patterns is easy. Anyone can do it. Changing your breathing starts with becoming aware of it.

BASIC BREATH

Your breath can be used to repel invading germs, to mend broken bones, to close wounds, to calm the mind, and to soothe upset emotions. Here are three affirmations you can use to activate the healing power in your breath:

- My breathing connects me to all parts of myself.
- Breath is my source, linking body, mind, and spirit.
- I now consciously breathe in the vital life force.

What breathing consciously does is to develop a communications link between consciousness and the unconscious, between body and mind, between spirit and psyche. Deep breathing is fundamental to the practice of all forms of oriental medicine, as is the healing power of relaxation—often taught through such oriental techniques as yoga and tai chi, and various forms of meditation.

This traditional worldview holds that the body was made by a powerful force that has been making life forms, including the human body, for eons. This force lives within you, and it contains millions of years of wisdom.

As a result of this point of view about the human body, in ancient societies the healers performed surgery, autopsied dead bodies, and investigated the functions of organs and tissues. However, their researches were guided by the principle of all-inclusive life, which asked the question, What causes this mass of flesh to function, and what gives an organ life? The answer was that the physical, corporeal body was not the complete story of life, and that underlying its life energy was the energy of life itself, a fundamental entity infuses the entire human being, and it is this that causes the body to have vitality, movement, and its various functions. This life force also provides the body with its own power to heal wounds, overcome disease, and face challenge and change.

Traditional medicine also took into account the *person*, the individual and his or her whole personality and history. Today, we are finally beginning to incorporate this knowledge into our approach to health and healing. Many studies now show that anger can contribute to heart disease and a range of other problems, including death, according to Dr. Mara Julius of the University of Michigan. And, in *Beyond Antibiotics*, Dr. Michael Schmidt states:

Anger and hostility eat away at the substance of the human psyche. The emotions foster an atmosphere of negativity that clouds every human endeavor. Researchers are increasingly showing a link between anger, hostility, and cynicism and the development of disease and premature death.

This is *not* a suggestion that we blame ourselves for getting sick. Most of the time we are not responsible for the negativity that comes our way, especially in childhood when many of the patterns that impact us negatively in later life are established. However, we *are* responsible for what we do with that negativity.

BREATHING HEALING ENERGY

This is a simple basic exercise designed to enable you to increase the vital force in your body in order to combat illness or effect healing. It can also be used anytime you are tired and need to refresh yourself. You can do this exercise almost anywhere—sitting quietly at home, in your car, on a train. (In the middle of a bustling city, I slip into a church, sit in a back pew, and breathe in energy.)

Relax and close your eyes. Tell yourself that you are now going to add vital energy every time you inhale deeply. Think of it as putting extra dollars into your energy bank for use whenever you need it. Realize that you are always surrounded by this vital healing force, that it sustains and nourishes you all the time, even when you are unaware of it.

Begin to breathe slowly and rhythmically, not altering your breath pattern but simply becoming aware of it. Now, begin to breathe deeply—slowly and deeply. As you inhale each breath, be aware of the energy coming into your body. Imagine it filling up all the cells of your body like you would fill a balloon by blowing air into it. Let the sense of being filled with energy spread throughout your body. Feel it energize your mind. Hold each breath for a few seconds while you imagine these results. Then, as you exhale feel the energy being retained within you. Let the breath go out smoothly and easily. Do not force or strain.

Abdominal, or diaphragmatic, breathing is "belly" breathing. When the air is taken in, the diaphragm contracts and the abdomen expands; when the air is exhaled, the reverse occurs. You can test yourself for abdominal breathing by laying your hand on your belly as you breathe. If it expands as you inhale, you are breathing with the diaphragm. If it flattens, you are breathing with the chest. To practice abdominal breathing, imagine that your in-breath is filling a balloon in your belly. When the balloon is full, exhale until you feel it is completely empty. Just a few of these deep abdominal breaths will bring relief from tension—and pain is half tension.

INSTANT MINI-RELAXATION

You can achieve instant relaxation simply by calling up the image you have created of your totally relaxed self. To do this, take a comfortable position and remember what it felt like to be completely relaxed. Your subconscious mind remembers everything. Take ten deep breaths, and when you have finished, you will be as completely relaxed as when you went through the entire relaxation process previously. Then, slowly and gently begin to breathe, counting ten breaths. If you like, for deeper relaxation, you can extend this to twenty breaths.

When you have finished the number of breaths you fixed in advance, you will feel relaxed and refreshed. Use this method frequently throughout the day. Relaxation transforms us physiologically as well as psychologically. It is also the gateway to the use of the other healing powers to be discussed.

We can refuse to continue in the negative patterns that have caused ill health. The experience of illness is a window of opportunity through which we can see clearly into our negative patterns and begin to transform them to conform to our true reality.

That the body also tends to symbolize illness through the affected parts has long been recognized by traditional medical practitioners, who insist that the *spirit* be treated along with the body. Some conditions, such as chronic stiffness, indicate something within that is restricted and needs to be released. Breast cancer is thought to be related to the nurturing a woman both gives and has received or—most often—has not received, and so on. Even accidents can be seen to have causal roots in the unconscious matrix if one looks closely enough. A broken arm can serve a psychological purpose.

A major factor in traditional medicine is *type*, each specific type being related to various parts of the body, the seasons, specific emotions, and appropriate herbs, as well as to one's self-image and general attitude toward life. These elements fundamentally influence our constitutional and immune system reactions on the physical plane. And because they are susceptible to being changed, we possess much more healing power than we know. Acting on this principle, traditional medicines around the world were intended to help mobilize the energy of the total organism in order to heal.

This idea of a universal life force was common among virtually all traditional peoples—in India it is called *prana*; in Japan, *ki*; in ancient Greece it was *pneuma*. All of the various terms actually refer to *breath*, which is considered to be the carrier of the life force.

Although Western medicine has largely ignored the benefits of conscious breathing, most Eastern philosophies teach that we live in a sea of vital energy—and that we

BREATHING RELAXATION

This is a simple technique that takes only a little time. Sit or lie down in a safe and comfortable spot with no distractions. Loosen any tight clothing; unbutton or untie anything that is restrictive on your body. Begin to breathe *consciously*, following your breath in and out of your lungs. Breathe in through the nostrils, out through the mouth. Pay full attention to your breath, in and out, in and out. Listen to the sound and feel the rhythmic pulsing of it. Continue this until you begin to feel calm and relaxed, a state usually signaled by the breath becoming slow and even.

You can deepen your relaxation using breath by imagining that you are breathing in *prana*, or the positive vital force of life, and exhaling all tension and negative feeling or experience. One way to do this is to choose two colors, one for the prana and one for the negative energy; see a stream of one color (positive) coming into your body as you inhale, and a stream of the other color (negative) flowing out of your body as you exhale. The colors white and black are easy to identify—white is the pure energy of light, and black represents any dark thoughts. But feel free to use any color that represents healing energy and release of negative energy to you. Don't worry if distracting thoughts arise. Let them float off (you can tell them you will attend to their needs later) like soap bubbles in the air and return to attending your breathing.

HERBS INSTEAD OF SURGERY

In China, cases that in the West would immediately be referred to a hospital for surgery are often treated herbally—80 percent of cases of acute appendicitis are routinely treated herbally instead of surgically.

A WOMAN'S HERBAL ANGEL

In Asia, Chinese angelica (*dang-qui*) has been used as a medicinal herb since ancient times. It was once thought to be the ideal herbal tonic for common gynecological problems. Traditional Chinese physicians today still recommend it for menstrual difficulties, as do Ayurvedic practitioners. American angelica was similarly used by Native Americans. Today, Chinese research suggests angelica may improve liver function, but this remains to be proven.

absorb and activate this with our breath. The Hindu yogi tradition calls this energy *prana*. Oriental mind-body balancing techniques, such as acupuncture and shiatsu, refer to this vital force as *Qi* (chi). The Hawaiian Huna tradition calls it *mana* (*mana loa* in its highest form). In the Hawaiian language, the word for "to think" is *mana-o*.

Not only is this subtle energy in the very air we breathe, it circulates through our bodies along specific channels called *meridians*. These are mapped along twelve courses, or channels, in the body. Imbalances in the energy flowing along these lines is believed to be the cause of illness.

It has been shown irrefutably what oriental medicine has always known—that tension and stress cause illness, from the minor aching of stiff muscles to heart and circulatory problems. Yet relaxation seems to evade us most of the time. Why? The answer is not completely clear, but clues can be found in our outlook on life. When we look upon life as an adversary or threat, we are in a perpetual state of "fight or flight." Instead of releasing the tension when danger is past, we store it; the retention results in a dangerous buildup that can bring on stress-related disease, such as high blood pressure, ulcers, and the like.

In the late 1960s, Harvard cardiologist Herbert Benson, M.D., was involved in some physiological tests on meditators. He discovered that relaxation methods, of which there are many, caused both psychological and physiological changes that served to counterbalance the body's response to "fight or flight." He called this the "relaxation response." Not a technique but a coordinated series of internal changes occurring when the mind and body become calm and tranquil, the relaxation response can be achieved by numerous means, such as deep breathing, muscle relaxation, meditation, visualization, and prayer. The simplest of these is called "focused meditation." Benson's tests showed that persons who simply sat quietly with their minds focused on a single word, idea, or thought could markedly change their physiology, decreasing metabolism, slowing heart and respiratory rates, and exhibiting brain waves of the alpha-theta pattern.

Benson showed that the relaxation response, no matter how it was achieved, caused bodily transformations: Heart rate, breathing rate, muscle tension, and oxygen consumption fall below resting

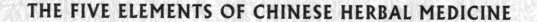

THE FIVE ELEMENTS OF CHINESE HERBAL MEDICINE

WOOD
Parts of the body: Liver, gallbladder, tendons, eyes
Season: Spring
Taste: Sour
Emotion: Anger

The "wood" element responds to sour herbs such as *shan zhu yu* and *wu wei zi*, which are generally astringent.

FIRE
Parts of the body: Heart, small intestine, tongue, blood vessels
Season: Summer
Taste: Bitter
Emotion: Joy

The "fire" element responds to bitter herbs, such as *dan shen* and *da huang* which are generally considered cooling.

EARTH
Parts of the body: Spleen, stomach, mouth, muscles
Season: Indian summer
Taste: Sweet
Emotion: Worry

The "earth" element responds to sweet herbs such as *gou qi zi* and *gan cao,* which are generally considered nutritional and tonifying.

METAL
Parts of the body: Lungs, large intestine, nose, skin
Season: Fall
Taste: Pungent
Emotion: Grief

The "metal" element responds to pungent herbs such as *bo he* and *ban xia,* considered to move *qi* through the blood.

WATER
Parts of the body: Kidneys, bladder, ears, hair, bones
Season: Winter
Taste: Salty
Emotion: Fear

The "water" element responds to salty herbs such as seaweeds, *qing dai* and *jin qian cao,* considered cooling.

PRINCIPLES OF CHINESE HERBAL MEDICINE

Oriental medicine includes a number of practices—including Chinese herbalism—that view the body as an energy vessel. Treatment is aimed at preventing or removing blockages of vital energy (called *qi* or *chi*).

Oriental medical practices are based on the traditional philosophies of China, Japan, Tibet, and related cultures and have existed for thousands of years.

Training varies depending on where in the world the practitioner lives or studied. Many practitioners trained in China have immigrated to the United States, and some Western doctors have gone to China to learn.

Oriental medicine is particularly appropriate for preventing disease, reducing chronic pain, rejuvenating the body, and healing deep-seated problems. Acupuncture can be used as an anesthetic in surgery.

levels; blood pressure can decrease; and the waking brain shifts into the slower patterns associated with reverie and daydreaming. These slightly altered states of consciousness promote healing in the same way sleep does.

In other studies, insomnia patients who elicited the relaxation response regularly were able to sleep better and return to normal sleep patterns; chronic pain patients were able to decrease their doctor visits by $1/3$; and patients with hypertension were able to lower their blood pressure. Also, psychologist Ann Webster, Ph.D., who teaches the relaxation response to patients with cancer and AIDS, has shown that these techniques reduce anticipatory nausea in those being treated with chemotherapy. Another Harvard study showed a 58 percent reduction of severe PMS symptoms.

Physical relaxation by itself may be an important adjunct to the healing process; consistent practice is a wonderful preventative measure.

Benson's work with meditators, who practiced an oriental system known as transcendental meditation, is in line with traditional systems, such as the Chinese and Greek, that hold that the body has the ability to cure itself of illness. In this view, the physician serves only to assist the body's own healing powers, as did the Greek physicians who served in the healing temples of Asklepios.

Chinese Herbal Medicine

Traditional Chinese herbal medicine has a history of nearly 5000 years. It employs a highly developed system, some of which is theoretical and philosophical, that determines the appropriate use of herbs for each case or occasion for which they are used. This system teaches that the causes of disease, illness, or any bodily or emotional dysfunction are various and that symptoms of the same dysfunction can vary with the individual.

As a result, the Chinese physician treats the *causes* underlying the problem, not the disease itself. It is this approach that allows even seemingly incurable conditions to be healed. Because Chinese herbalists are taught to recognize the various patterns of the causes of disease and are trained in the specific qualities and uses of each herb in their vast pharmacological repertoire, they focus on what is happening with the *person* rather than on symptom removal.

For example, the working of any single organ is seen within the context of the whole—an eye problem may be seen as a symptom of an underlying imbalance in the liver. Treatment would include an examination of the person's entire life—what he or she generally ate, family and other relationships, working habits. A headache might be diagnosed as including liver congestion, stomach upset, tension, or some organ weakness, which would vary according to the individual's current state of health. Therefore, a combination of herbs might be included in the treatment, chosen specifically for that individual. This holistic approach clearly differs significantly from the Western method of prescribing aspirin (from the herbal source willow bark) or a similar NSAID for everyone suffering from headache.

The Chinese healer would look for the effects on the person's *qi* (vital energy) of all the components of his or her life, and treat accordingly, as different herbs would be used to address different causes of the same symptom. By working to strengthen the underlying life force while at the same time providing symptomatic relief, the Chinese healer is enlisting the body's own healing mechanisms as an ally in overcoming the disorder.

To do this, traditional Chinese medicine includes daily participation in such movements as *tai chi chuan* and *qi gong* as well as the use of medicinal herbs and the development of a healthy set of habits governing life. Much Chinese medicine is *preventative*—in contrast to the type of allopathic medicine practiced in the Western world—and the Chinese people use herbs on a regular basis, either daily or weekly. They might drink a special herbal soup to aid their adjustment to seasonal, emotional, hormonal, job, or environmental changes, for example, when moving to a new location.

The long history of Chinese herbal medicine includes texts that are still studied and followed; while much has been added

CHINESE TONICS

A particular category of Chinese herbs, tonics, has proven most effective. Tonic herbs are divided into four subcategories: for energy (*qi*), for blood, for warming and activating (*yang*), and for cooling and moistening (*yin*).

A VERY ANCIENT REMEDY

Ginseng has been in continuous use in China for over 4000 years. The first written reference to it appears in *Shen-Nung Pen Ts'ao Ching*. A revision in the 5th century adds that ginseng is for "repairing the five viscera, quieting the spirit, curbing the emotions, stopping agitation, removing the noxious influence, brightening the eyes, enlightening the mind, and increasing the wisdom." It also adds that "continuous use leads to longevity and light weight."

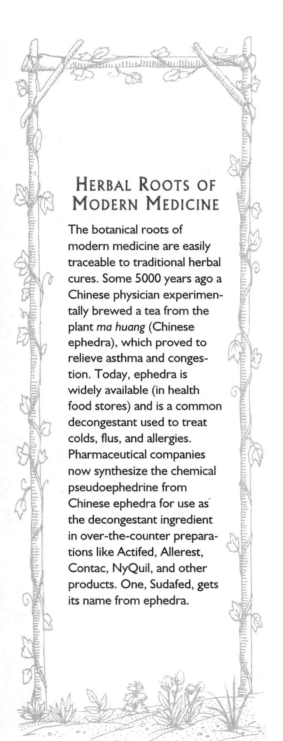

HERBAL ROOTS OF MODERN MEDICINE

The botanical roots of modern medicine are easily traceable to traditional herbal cures. Some 5000 years ago a Chinese physician experimentally brewed a tea from the plant *ma huang* (Chinese ephedra), which proved to relieve asthma and congestion. Today, ephedra is widely available (in health food stores) and is a common decongestant used to treat colds, flus, and allergies. Pharmaceutical companies now synthesize the chemical pseudoephedrine from Chinese ephedra for use as the decongestant ingredient in over-the-counter preparations like Actifed, Allerest, Contac, NyQuil, and other products. One, Sudafed, gets its name from ephedra.

over the years, almost nothing has been deleted. Herbs are central to treatment, and treatment is related to the elements, of which in Chinese philosophy there are five (not four, as in the Greek model discussed in Chapter 1).

This theory of elements is used to explain every interaction between humans and their environments, and each element has specific associations. For good health to prevail, the elements must be in harmony. In addition, the Chinese principle of *yin* and *yang*, already discussed, is a major part of this theoretical systems, and any imbalance between the two can affect health and well-being. Different parts of the body are considered to be either predominately *yin* or *yang*.

The five elements form a network of relationships, and various herbs can be linked to the model in various ways—the taste of the herb might suggest the bodily organ for which it is an appropriate treatment.

How Chinese Herbs Are Prescribed

The Chinese usually prescribe herbs in standardized formulae, of which there are several thousand in regular use! These formulae may be adjusted somewhat, depending on the individual patient and what is bothering him or her. Some formulae include just a couple of herbs; others contain as many as twenty. In the Chinese view, the interaction between the herbs themselves is as important as the interaction between the patient and the herbal remedy. Unfortunately for the non-Chinese, or the layperson, this system—though it often results in dramatic therapeutic effects—is not subject to the Western scientific approach. In fact, it generally defies all attempts at rational scientific examination.

The form in which Chinese herbs are administered also varies—there are pills and powders, just as Westerners use, but the most common form is in soups, which are decoctions brewed at home according to the physician's instructions, or as family remedies. Sometimes the medicinal herbs are cooked with rice and eaten as a therapeutic meal.

The following is a list of 31 of the most popular Chinese herbs, compiled by Earl Mindell in his *Herb Bible*, that are

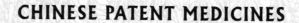

CHINESE PATENT MEDICINES

The following Chinese patent medicines, manufactured by Chinese pharmaceutical companies, may be available through American sources such as Elixir:

- CHIN KOO TIEH SHANG WAN (Tientsin Drug Manufacturing, Tientsin, China)—used to treat chronic arthritis swelling, inflammation, and pain

- CORYDALIS YANHUSUS (Chongqing Chinese Medicine Factory, Chongqing Sichuan, China)—whose label states it "breaks obstruction of energy and blood;" an analgesic

- TIN TZAT TO CHUNG (Shan sai Hang Lam Medicine Manufactory, Hong Kong)—used as "relief for arthritic pains and rheumatisms" and to enhance circulation

- ZHENG GU SHI (Yulin Drug Factory, Kwangsi, China)—labeled as a "topical liniment for aching joints"

- ARTHRITIC is a formula in the "Jade Herbals" line from East Earth Herb, Inc. (P.O. Box 2802, Eugene, OR 97402.) Call toll free at 800-827-4372 for information about this and other American-made Chinese herbal medicines.

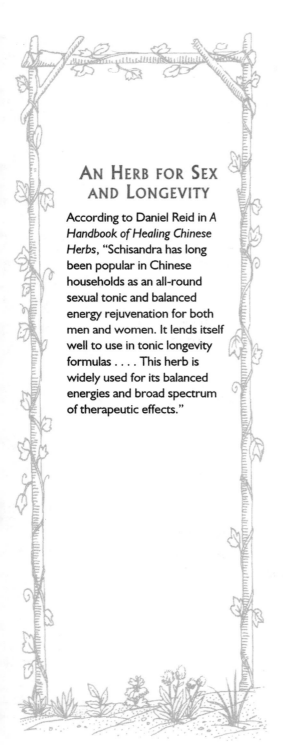

AN HERB FOR SEX AND LONGEVITY

According to Daniel Reid in *A Handbook of Healing Chinese Herbs,* "Schisandra has long been popular in Chinese households as an all-round sexual tonic and balanced energy rejuvenation for both men and women. It lends itself well to use in tonic longevity formulas . . . . This herb is widely used for its balanced energies and broad spectrum of therapeutic effects."

currently available in the United States. Some of these may be available at health food stores or through mail order catalogs; others may be found only in special herbal shops—usually located in the Chinatowns of cities with large Asian populations, such as New York and San Francisco. Some of the herbs listed have more than one Chinese name because to variations in dialect and not all of them will be familiar to Westerners. Where available, English names are given in parentheses.

TOP THIRTY CHINESE HERBS
MUXU or ZIMU (Alfalfa)
BA DAN XING REN (Almond)
LU HUI (Aloe vera)
LUOLE (Basil)
DOU FU-TOFU (Bean curd)
YE JU (Chrysanthemum)
PU GONG YING (Dandelion)
HU SUAN (Garlic)
GAN JIANG (Ginger)
REN SHEN (Ginseng)
GAN CAO (Licorice)
FAN MU GUA (Papaya)
FAN JIA (Hot pepper)
MI DIE XIANG (Rosemary)
HUANG CHI (Astragalus)
BUPLERUM or CH'AI HU
LU RONG (Deer antler)
DONG QUAI or TANG KUEI
DON SEN or TANG SHEN
MA HUANG (Ephedra)
HO SHOU or FO-TI
DA T'SAO (Jujube date)
GAY GEE (Lycii)
PAI SHU
PLATYCODON or JIE ENG
PUERARIA or KO KEN
REHMANNIA or SOK-DAY-SANG-DAY
SCHIZANDRA FRUCTUS or SCHIZANDRA CHINENSIS
SILERIS or FANG-FENG

Because the use of Chinese herbs requires (1) determination of the individual's constitution, (2) evaluation of the nature of the disease, and (3) the choice of herbs that match both the *qi* (energy) of the person and the *qi* of the disease, using Chinese herbs is a complex matter. The reader is advised to consult with either a Chinese herbal practitioner or a licensed Chinese acupuncturist with herbal knowledge. Self-prescription of Chinese herbs is not advised, but the person wanting to learn more can refer to a number of books on the subject, such as *A Handbook of Healing Chinese Herbs* by Daniel Reid.

Ayurvedic Medicine

Legend tells us that the Indian traditional system of health and healing, Ayurveda—which is considered to be the knowledge of achieving long life—was presented as a gift to a great Hindu rishi, or wise man, by the god Indra. The word *Ayurveda* is derived from two Indian words: *ayur* (life) and *veda* (knowledge). Thus, ayur-veda means "knowledge of life," or "knowledge of how to live the life that one is given by the gods." In this system, as in other traditional systems, illness is seen as an imbalance of the vital forces and the treatments with herbs—and strict dietary means—are used to restore equilibrium.

No one knows just how long ago Indra gave the knowledge to the rishi, but scholars do know that the Ayurvedic system dates back to at least the 5th century B.C.E. and that is is based on the ancient philosophical and spiritual texts of India known as the Vedas, of which there are several different ones written at different periods of Indian history.

In the Hindu Ayurveda system—as in the Chinese and Greek systems—human health is seen within a cosmic context—as an extension of the life of the creator, or original source of cosmic consciousness. The Indian religious pantheon of gods and goddesses is vast and complex, but it is based essentially upon a cre-

HELPFUL RESOURCES

For information about Chinese acupuncturists who are also qualified as Chinese herbalists, contact the American Association of Acupuncture and Oriental Medicine, 433 Front Street, Catasauqua, PA 18032. Or call 610-433-2448.

&~&

Elixir is the name of a Los Angeles shop specializing in Chinese herbs and Chinese medicine. It has a qualified herbalist on staff available for telephone consultation, which means that anyone anywhere can call Elixir and get advice on using Chinese herbs. Customers can buy single herbs to create self-designed programs or herbal combinations for specific needs—the traditional Chinese practitioner's method of prescribing herbs. Call 888-486-6427. You can also request their free catalog.

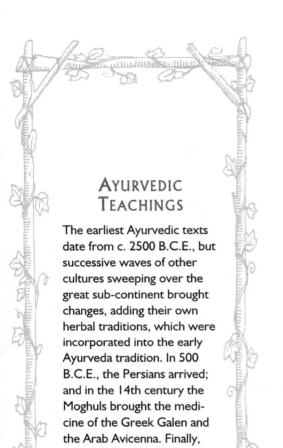

AYURVEDIC TEACHINGS

The earliest Ayurvedic texts date from c. 2500 B.C.E., but successive waves of other cultures sweeping over the great sub-continent brought changes, adding their own herbal traditions, which were incorporated into the early Ayurveda tradition. In 500 B.C.E., the Persians arrived; and in the 14th century the Moghuls brought the medicine of the Greek Galen and the Arab Avicenna. Finally, the British, during their occupation of India, closed down the Ayurvedic schools in 1833. This did not obliterate the Ayurvedic tradition; it simply went underground where it continued to be practiced in secret, just as the "herb wives" of England kept alive their herbal medicine tradition.

ation myth that holds that from a single, unified and cosmic consciousness, two forces, once united, split and emerged separately. These are called *Shiva* and *Shakti* and represent the male and female principles, respectively, just as *yang* and *yin* do in the Chinese system.

These two forces combine to create all the multiple forms of being, physical and nonphysical through the manifestation of a life force, called *prana*, which is the animating power of life in every living being. It is also the basis of healing. The belief is that health is based upon one's personal relationship with cosmic consciousness; a healer serves only as a conduit to re-establish harmony between the sick individual and the universal life force, doing so by balancing the forces within each person that correspond to the universal forces.

As with the Greek and Chinese systems, Ayurveda holds that there are elements that are responsible for the composition of the life force. In India, as in China, there are five elements: earth, water, fire, air, and ether. Each of the five elements is responsible for the individual senses and their functions. Fire is associated with the eyes and seeing; air governs touch and the skin; water, taste and the tongue; earth, smell and the nose; and ether, hearing and the ear.

Of course, these elements and their relationships to the human body are not seen as being material; they are more metaphorical categories that are used to describe aspects of the human physical body and its functions. Fire, for example, rules the function of digestion, and the body's digestive system can be likened to a "crucible" that heats and dissolves the food taken in, converting it to nutrients.

The earth element is related to all of the mineral substances from which the body is made; calcium, for example, is needed in the formation of muscle, bones, teeth, and cartilage. Earth also represents the body's solid waste.

Water is the element that represents all of the body's fluids—blood, mucus, lymph, hormones, semen, urine, and so on. As such, water is related to the genitals and reproductive processes.

Ether, a nebulous nothingness that fills the void between solid objects was also part of the Greek system. It is the principle of form, and from ether the body gets its design. Ether is

LOTUS MEDITATION

Prepare for this meditation by choosing a quiet place where you can be alone and comfortable for half an hour. Breathe slowly and deeply several times and allow your body to relax completely. Imagine yourself a seed at the bottom of a deep pool where all is dark and tranquil. Feel yourself begin to put out roots into the nourishing bottom and anchor yourself there. Next, feel a stem begin to grow up and out of you, reaching toward the light above. Feel it move through the abyssal water until it breaks the surface. Then, feel yourself putting out new little leaves on the surface of the water, stretching in all directions.

As these leaves grow larger and stronger, feel yourself growing into the bud of a beautiful lotus. Let this bud rest on the surface, in the light, for a few minutes and then—slowly—begin to open up your petals, one by one, until you have unfurled a glorious blossom, fully opened and gently floating on its undulant stem, but firmly rooted in the earth at the bottom of the pond. Feel the light on your petals, soak up the warmth of the sun, breathe in the cool of the air. Say, *I open to my inner healing powers. I release and let go all constraints, restrictions, limits.*

Remain with this feeling of being totally, safely, and completely open for as long as the feeling lasts. When it begins to fade, *slowly* return to waking consciousness by breathing gently and easily, continuing to feel yourself as open to your inner possibilities for healing.

Rest quietly until you feel yourself retracting into the bud state. Now that your lotus self has blossomed fully, you know you can always open when you wish. You do not need to be fully open all of the time—you can rest in the bud state, or even return to the seed state to gather new force. The goal is to be *able* to open fully to the transformative process of self-healing.

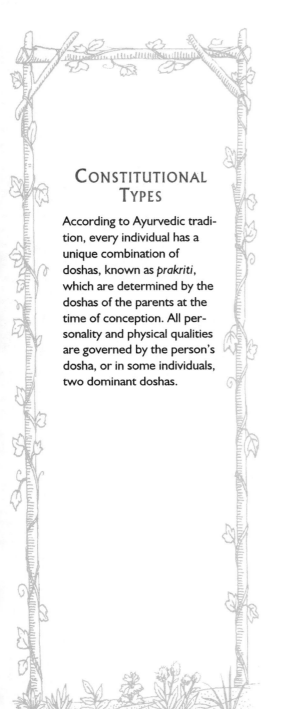

CONSTITUTIONAL TYPES

According to Ayurvedic tradition, every individual has a unique combination of doshas, known as *prakriti*, which are determined by the doshas of the parents at the time of conception. All personality and physical qualities are governed by the person's dosha, or in some individuals, two dominant doshas.

a sort of invisible glue that holds the whole system together. (From *ether* we get the word *ethereal* to mean something that is neither here nor there while being everywhere.)

Ayruvedic medicine emphasizes a holistic approach—as does the Chinese system—by using remedies appropriate for the individual and by considering the mind and spirit as well as the body. It incorporates herbs, nutrition, meditation, rest, exercise, massage, yoga, and thus helps the patient unleash his or her self-healing powers.

A key component of Ayurveda is meditation, which helps us become grounded in our connection with the wholeness of nature. Ayurveda recognizes that many of our ailments are a result of constriction and repression; for example, stomach cramps are produced by fear and anxiety, and rheumatic stiffness symbolizes an unbending attitude.

In other words, the inner pattern of stiffness and constraint works itself out bodily, becoming innervation, constricted movements and behaviors, and illness, especially chronic pain. Closing one's self off to the gamut of humanity's multiplicity means living in a state of perennial constriction and isolation, with concomitant results.

Problems of the heart, for example, are seen to be as much of a spiritual as a pathological issue, because the heart is the seat of the *atman*, or Divine Self. The heart would in this view be seen as "closed" to the divine energy, or *prana*, and meditation would be an effective tool to open the heart and heal the body. For example, a pattern of dogmatic self-righteousness and emotional denial can concur with cardiac and circulatory malfunction, such as the aptly named "hardening of the arteries," which often precedes cardiac arrest.

One of the primary tenets of Ayurveda is that the best way to fight disease is to strengthen the host—that illness results from underlying imbalances that occur when the individual goes against the body's own innate intelligence. By paying proper attention and respecting Nature's laws, Ayurveda tells us that the body will regain balance and restore itself.

Opening ourselves to the vast possibilities inherent in our own natures releases great healing power. If we are to access all available means to treat ourselves when we fall ill, it is important to develop emotional openness to our own healing abilities. Unfortunately, many of us have lost touch with our body's nature by closing down our emotional responses, and illness is the price of neglect.

The Theory of the Doshas

The *doshas* are the cornerstone of Ayurvedic medicine—once again, as in Chinese and Greek systems, based on type. The theory holds that the doshas are three constantly fluctuating energies that define all things in the universe: *vata, pitta*, and *kapha*. Each dosha is made of a combination of two of the five elements (already discussed) of the Ayurvedic system:

Vata is formed from air and ether; pitta is made up of fire and water; kapha is a combination of water and earth. Each has distinctive qualities that can be recognized in human beings and in the environment. In humans, there are definite descriptions of each type (although it is rare for a human being to exactly fit any one type). These are:

Pitta describes a person with an average body, strong intellect, a robust appetite, and a determined personality. The physical appearance of a pitta type includes reddish hair and/or skin (freckles) and poor eyesight, requiring the wearing of eyeglasses. Anger is the emotion related to pitta. Treatments for pitta types include "cooling" herbs, moderate exercise, avoidance of direct sun, and hot baths or saunas. Pitta types are said to be vulnerable to infections, ulcers, jaundice, heartburn, acne, herpes, cancer sores, and Crohn's disease.

Vata describes a person who may be very tall or very short and who does not gain weight no matter how much food is consumed. Vata types seem to run on nervous energy and tend to sleep and eat irregularly. They are creative and restless by nature but suffer from fear and anxiety. Ayurvedic treatment would include light exercise, a rigid routine for sleeping and waking, meditation, steam baths, and massage. Vatas are said to be susceptible to manic-depression, heart palpitations, tremors, insomnia, dry skin, constipation, sciatica, and muscle weakness.

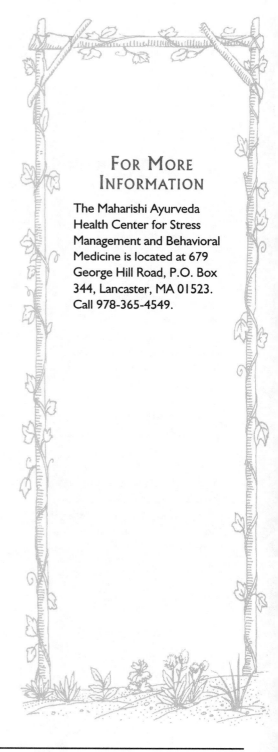

FOR MORE INFORMATION

The Maharishi Ayurveda Health Center for Stress Management and Behavioral Medicine is located at 679 George Hill Road, P.O. Box 344, Lancaster, MA 01523. Call 978-365-4549.

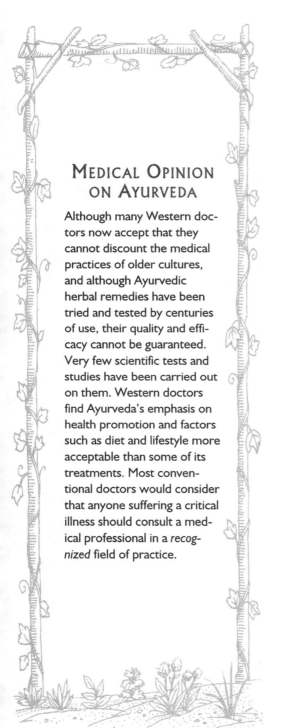

MEDICAL OPINION ON AYURVEDA

Although many Western doctors now accept that they cannot discount the medical practices of older cultures, and although Ayurvedic herbal remedies have been tried and tested by centuries of use, their quality and efficacy cannot be guaranteed. Very few scientific tests and studies have been carried out on them. Western doctors find Ayurveda's emphasis on health promotion and factors such as diet and lifestyle more acceptable than some of its treatments. Most conventional doctors would consider that anyone suffering a critical illness should consult a medical professional in a *recognized* field of practice.

Kapha describes a person with a large body and even temperament. Although the kapha type gains weight easily, they can go for long periods without food, having great stamina. They tend to move slowly and learn slowly but have great retentive power. Ayurvedic treatment for kaphas include aerobic exercise, deep massage, using a firm mattress, saunas, and a limited intake of water daily.

The Practice of Ayurvedic Medicine

The use of herbal medicines is an important part of Ayurvedic practice. Two areas of focus that the Ayurvedic herbal formulae address are digestion and emotional well-being.

Ayurvedic remedies are made from up to 20 different herbs, minerals, and vegetables. They should be prescribed by a qualified practitioner, as self-diagnosis is not wise for the treatment of any serious condition.

Ayurveda is widely practiced in India alongside Western, conventional medicine, and, following Indian independence in 1947, Ayurveda experienced a revival in India. Today, a central council monitors its training and practice, and colleges offer a degree in Ayurveda, which includes courses of basic study of Western medicine.

There are a limited number of practitioners of Ayurveda in the United States, some of whom have trained in India. However, it is important for Americans to realize that *Ayurveda is not a licensed medical practice anywhere in the United States*.

In the United States, Ayurveda is mainly practiced as part of "Maharishi Ayur-Ved," a system established by followers of the yogi Maharishi Mahesh (whose organization teaches transcendental meditation). Maharishi Mahesh, along with his former associate, Deepak Chopra, the popular Indian "guru" and writer, has largely been responsible for focusing attention on Ayurveda in this country.

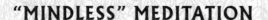

"MINDLESS" MEDITATION

Here is a meditation devised to put you into a state of mind that can lead to real rest. To do this meditation—which is really not a meditation at all in any formal sense—recline or lie down comfortably when you can be alone and uninterrupted for an hour. Turn lights down or off and eliminate outside noises and distractions. Close your eyes and let yourself experience the silence around you, then move inward and find a place of silence inside. Let yourself stay in this place as long as you feel comfortable. Begin to follow your breath without trying to alter it. Just feel the quiet rhythm of your SELF. As you do this, let your mind wander wherever it wants to go, like a puppy let outside for an airing. Follow it if you wish, to see what interests it, but make no judgments. Think of your mind as a butterfly lighting on one flower, now on another, gathering nectar. Don't push or move your mind in any particular direction. *Let it go where it wants*. That is the key here. So much meditation tries to harness the mind, tether it like a goat on a rope as bait for large game. Don't do that. As your mind is given the freedom to roam here and there, to *play* at will, it will lead you to your place of rest.

THE RAIN FOREST TRAGEDY

Many rich and unexplored sources of medicinal plant knowledge are being eradicated through the heedless and wanton destruction of the world's remaining rain forests. Vast tracts of the Amazonian rain forests are being broken up and their native tribes dispersed. This is a tragedy of major proportions not only in terms of humans being displaced but also in terms of the permanent loss of invaluable and irreplaceable information about thousands of local medicinal plant species, now being condemned to extinction. This destruction is taking place despite the fact that it was from native tribes living in their own habitats that Western medicine learned the plant sources of most of its commonly used drugs—ipecac and quinine, for example.

Popular Ayurvedic herbs include the following:

Amalaki is used to treat eating disorders and normalize bowel functions.

Ashwagandha is prescribed for a reactive type of depression and t heal broken bones, and is claimed to have beneficial effects on cancer, arthritis, ulcers, hypertension, and stress.

Boswellia serrata is used for a variety of intestinal complaints and has been recommended for colitis.

Brahmi is used to relieve anxiety and as a treatment for epilepsy and leprosy.

Coleus forskohlii is claimed to achieve reduction of excess atherosclerosis-causing platelet clumping, improve heart-muscle contraction, to relax the arteries and other smooth muscles, reduce histamine release; increase insulin release; and improve thyroid function.

Gotu kola is used to reduce levels of anxiety and mental weariness

Guduchi is a traditional remedy for diabetes and ulcers.

Guggul is used to lower blood cholesterol levels.

Neem is used for blood disorders, eye diseases, fevers, skin diseases, and ulcers.

Sarsaparilla acts as a blood purifier and is used to treat fever, skin diseases, genitourinary conditions, chronic coughs, and poor appetite

Senna, mentioned in the *Rig Veda* as a treatment for constipation, i today an ingredient in many commercial laxatives such as Fletcher's Castoria and Innerclean Herbal Laxative.

Shanka Puspi is used as a mild painkiller and to treat anxiety.

Sida cordifolia is used for spasmodic coughs and asthma, to treat urinary infections, and as an antibacterial, antifungal, and antiviral agent.

Vacha is said to have a calming effect on the body and is reputed to be an aphrodisiac.

Herbs from the World's Rain Forests

Leslie Taylor, in *Herbal Secrets of the Rainforest*, states the following:

It is estimated that nearly half of the world's estimated ten million species of plants, animals, and microorganisms will be destroyed or severely threatened over the next quarter of a century due to rainforest deforestation. Harvard's Pulitzer Prize winner biologist Edward O. Wilson estimates that we are losing 137 plant, animal, and insect species every single day. That's 50,000 species a year! Why should we in the United States be concerned about the destruction of distant tropical rainforests? Because rainforest plants are complex chemical storehouses that contain many undiscovered biodynamic compounds with unrealized potential for use in modern medicine. We can gain access to these materials only if we study and conserve the species that contain them. Rainforests currently provide sources for $\frac{1}{4}$ of today's medicines, and 70 percent of the plants found to have anticancer properties are found only in the rainforest. The rainforest and its immense undiscovered biodiversity hold the key to unlocking tomorrow's cures for devastating diseases. How many cures for devastating disease have we already lost?

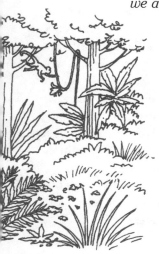

The number of potentially useful medicinal plants growing in the world's rain forests is estimated to be in the thousands. There is no doubt human health would benefit from the understanding and application of these plants. Future years could see the discovery of cures for many of today's serious diseases—such as AIDS and cancer to name only two—that have defeated researchers' efforts to find cures. Such is the enormous potential value of the herbs and plants of the rain forests that there are those who

SHAMAN SECRETS

In the preface to his *Medicinal Plants of East Africa*, Jo Kokwaro commented that native plant knowledge is jealously guarded from outsiders, traditionally passed on by the medicine men only to a chosen successor. He said he had to use bribes and other methods to gain information because "a few people categorically refuse to reveal their secrets."

RAIN FOREST INFORMATION

For more information on preserving what's left of the precious resources in our rapidly disappearing rain forests around the world, write Rainforest Alliance, 270 Lafayette Street, Suite 512, New York, NY 10012.

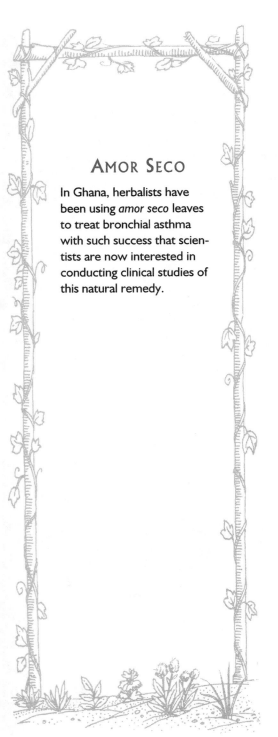

Amor Seco

In Ghana, herbalists have been using *amor seco* leaves to treat bronchial asthma with such success that scientists are now interested in conducting clinical studies of this natural remedy.

believe *all* future curative medicines will be discovered in them, changing the face of Western medicine forever.

As much as we would like to see immediate results from explorations of rain forest plants—before any more extinction of species occurs!—there is no choice but to proceed slowly. We cannot expect to have a river of rain forest remedies just come pouring out of the jungles.

The indigenous peoples of the rain forests and other remote places on the earth seem quite satisfied to simply utilize methods for the location and preparation of their native plants that have been passed down from generation to generation in accordance with custom—not only medical but also social and religious ways.

Medicinal Plants of the Rain Forest

There are literally thousands of rain forest plants that would make wonderful additions to the world's pharmacopoeia yet, only a few have actually made their way to that status despite the current obvious phenomenon of drug companies rushing to South America and the South Pacific Islands—most often under the sponsorship of the National Cancer Institute—in desperate search of novel compounds.

This trend includes dozens of North American herbalists who are tagging along in their wake. Though their motives are not clear, they do seem to be more interested in knowledge than in profit-taking. Video clips of some of these exploration teams have shown the drug seekers gazing in awe at the effective application of rain forest medicinals by local shamans and herbal medicine men. The researchers, quite stupefied by what they are witnessing, are in a heat to rush back to their laboratories to discover how the remedies they have seen in action really "work." What's in them, and what does it do?

The need for haste is not in doubt. However, it would seem that the primary task of all concerned—especially drug companies, who, while ironically disparaging herbal medicine, are dependent on herbal sources for their patented and profitable drugs—would be to show respect to the plants themselves and to the local people who know about their uses.

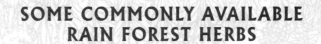

SOME COMMONLY AVAILABLE
RAIN FOREST HERBS

Following are some of the most important healing medicinal plants, along with descriptions of their uses, as listed in *Herbal Secrets of the Rainforest* by Leslie Taylor. You can learn more by reading *Kava: Medicine Hunting in Paradise* by Chris Kilham, the founder of Cowboy Medicine Expeditions, through which he conducts research on medicinal plants around the world.

ACEROLA—Contains vitamin C. Promotes a healthy circulatory system.

ALCACHOFRA (Artichoke)—Detoxifies the liver. Digestive stimulant. Eat whole vegetable or buy standard extract from health food store.

ANNATO—Used as a natural food coloring agent; also used in cheese and cheese products. May have other health benefits.

BOLDO—Detoxifies the liver; rids liver of fat. Promotes healthy bile flow.

CAT'S CLAW—Aids intestinal immune system and chronic arthritis.

CATUABA—Aphrodisiac; used to promote hormone regulation.

DAMIANA—Used for hormone regulation in men and women.

GUARANA—Promotes health and energy.

MACA—Antifatigue; for hormone regulation; general health tonic.

MUIRA PUAMA—Relieves stress; regulates hormones; promotes healthy central nervous system; general health tonic.

PAU D'ARCO—Fights fungus infections and viral infections; stimulates immune system.

STEVIA—Regulates blood sugar. (Popular sweetener because it contains no calories.) Regulates hormones.

SUMA—Regulates female hormones; strengthens immune system; aids in regulation of cholesterol. Also used as general health tonic. Also known as Brazilian Ginseng.

YERBA MATE—Contains vitamin C; relieves upset stomach; general health tonic.

NONPROFIT RAIN FOREST ORGANIZATIONS

Amazon Center for Environmental Education and Research
Ten Environs Park
Helena, Alabama 35080
800-255-8206
APECA
12 South Main Street, Suite 302
West Hartford, Connecticut 06107
860-232-6971
Web site: *http://www.apeca.org*
Founded in 1993, APECA began as a floating health clinic, delivering medical services to the remote Amazon River villages. It has since established programs in health education, nutrition, natural medicine, and sanitation.

Center for World Indigenous Studies
Post Office Box 2574
Olympia, Washington 98507
Fax: 360-956-2574
Web site: *http://www.halcyon.com/FWDP/cwisinfo.html*
The center is devoted to the understanding and appreciation of the ideas and knowledge of indigenous peoples.

Conservation International
1015 18th Street, NW, Suite 1000
Washington, D.C. 20036
202-429-5660

Web site: *http://www.conservation.org/clap.htm*
This organization promotes biodiversity conservation in rain forests and other endangered ecosystems worldwide.

The Rainforest Action Network
301 Broadway, Suite A
San Francisco, California 94133
Web site: *http://www.ran.org*
The network works to protect the Earth's rain forests and the rights of their inhabitants.

Rainforest Conservation Fund
2038 North Carl, Suite 233
Chicago, Illinois 60614
312-975-7571
The fund conducts various projects in the Amazon for the sustainable harvesting of rain forest plants, fruits, and nuts.

Rainforest Preservation Foundation
Post Office Box 820308
Ft. Worth, Texas 76182
817-222-1155
This organization buys endangered rain forest land in Brazil and places it in trust.

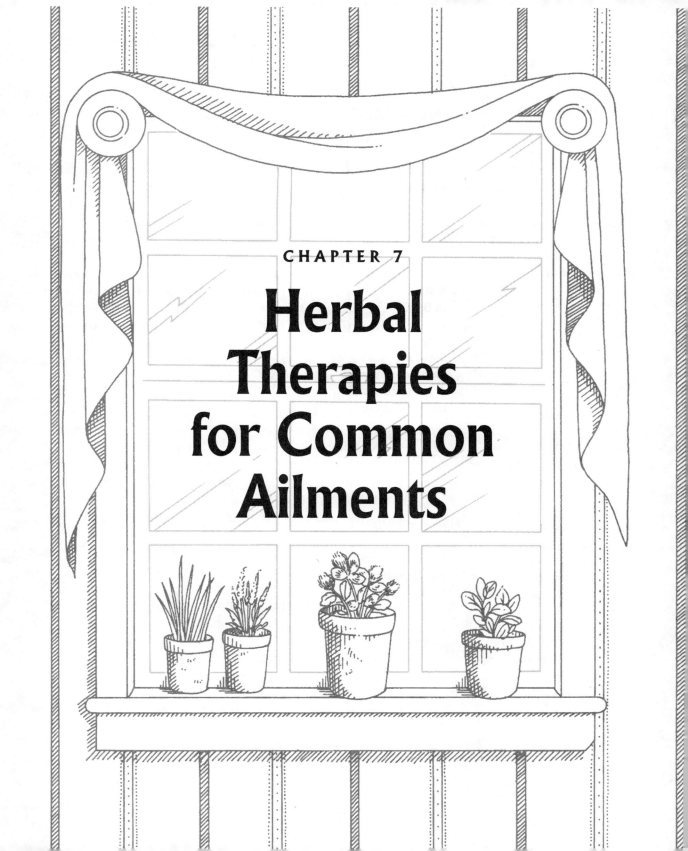

CHAPTER 7

Herbal Therapies for Common Ailments

PLANTS AS PHARMACISTS

As research into the actions of plant chemicals progresses, it may give credibility to one of the bases of "sympathetic magic," the notion that a plant's physiology provides clues to its medicinal use. An example of the many constituents of herbs containing certain chemicals with useful actions for the plant that are also beneficial to human users is that of tannin, which is contained in the leaves of certain plants. Tannin and other bitter chemicals deter insect predators. In herbal medicines, they act to promote the healing of wounds.

The reason plant substances may have a comparable effect on human chemistry is because all on Earth has evolved from a common biological ancestry. We are all related—plant, animal, human (and perhaps mineral) kingdoms. Research has shown that some of the most basic elements in the cells of human bodies share properties with those in plants.

Herbal healing exemplifies universal truth at its highest level. It is both a science and an art, with qualities we would all like to represent, and the ones we value most in ourselves. In a very grasping world, they are always giving. They show us how health care ought to be . . . conscious of the whole person, easy to use, gentle, safe, inexpensive, always available, and able to handle any problem.

—LINDA RECTOR PAGE, N.D., PH.D.

Medical herbalism is an inexact term. To some extent, herbal remedies overlap with conventional medicine; many of our over-the-counter and prescription drugs, such as aspirin and digitalis, are based on plant derivatives. However, medical herbalism differs in important ways from both home herbal remedies of the folk tradition and modern medicine.

A major difference is that medical herbalism refers to the use of whole herbs, on the basis that the active principles are better utilized by the body if they are not isolated from other organic substances that occur in the same plant. A second important difference is that many herbs are used to treat deep-seated nutritional or biochemical problems or deficiencies in individual patients, making them much more effective for a particular person, but also requiring more time to work than conventional drugs.

It is difficult to scientifically test and evaluate the medical use of herbs in the laboratory. These plants are complex, which may be why they have such a dramatic effect on human physiology. All living things, including humans, are composed of families of related organic compounds. Therefore the proteins, enzymes, sugars, vitamins, minerals, and even toxic substances found in plants will affect the human system by relating to similar substances found in the body, a fact that may account for the "sympathetic" concept already discussed.

Frequently a plant chemical when applied to a human system will mimic its own usual reaction inside the plant from which it originated. A classic example of this reaction is that

Coriander

of antibiotics, which in plants evolved to ward off attacks by specific bacteria and fungi; these substances act the same way in animals. Thus, it appears that there may be similarly transferable processes between plants and humans.

There are also many subtle similarities between plant and animal biochemistry, beyond the more direct relationship already described. For example, human sex hormones have been discovered in yeast and certain fungi. Several plants contain compounds in themselves that resemble those found naturally in humans, such as the endorphins that inhibit pain.

The World Health Organization (WHO) is making efforts all over the globe to safeguard the kind of medicine, called "folk," or "traditional," on which the bulk of the world's population depends, just as it has for eons. Their continuing fieldwork among indigenous peoples is of great value—and urgently needed. Plant species are disappearing at an alarming rate and can never be replaced. A vast amount of herbal knowledge gained over the centuries is being lost with the disappearance of the forest habitats—especially the rain forests—and the displacement of their inhabitants, whose information about the properties of native and local herbs and plants is often stored in memory, not in written records.

Common Ailments and Herbs Appropriate to Their Treatment

See Chapter 5 for specifics on each herb.

Allergies—Alfalfa, Burdock, Comfrey, Echinacea, Goldenseal, and Ma Huang

Anorexia Nervosa—Chamomile, Dandelion, Kelp, Ladies Slipper, Licorice, Passionflower, Skullcap, Red Clover, Wild Yam, and Yellow Dock

Arthritis—Alfalfa, Devil's Claw, Echinacea, White Willow, and Yucca

Asthma—Alfalfa, Asthma Weed, Capsicum, Chlorophyll, Cacara Sagrada, Comfrey, Fenugreek, Garlic, Hops, Licorice, Ma Huang (Ephedra) and Slippery Elm

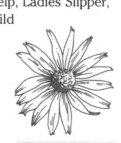

Echinacea

RECOMMENDED READING FOR ARTHRITIS SUFFERERS

The recently published book, *The Arthritis Bible*, by Craig Weatherby and Leonid Gordin, M.D., is a comprehensive guide to alternative therapies—including a thorough discussion of herbal treatments and the scientific evidence relating to them.

ATTENTION ASTHMA SUFFERERS

Chinese medicine often associated asthma with weak kidney energy and a failure of proper *qi* circulation. Kidney tonics such as gui zhi could be appropriate in treatment.

Important: Severe asthma can be life-threatening and requires medical help. Chronic asthmatics should seek professional medical advice before stopping orthodox treatment.

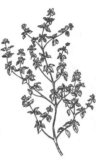

Thyme

AH-CHOO! COLDS AND INFLUENZA

Colds and flu are generally considered to be due to viral or bacterial infections and often associated with stress, fatigue, depression, and excess cold or heat. We all know the symptoms: fever, muscle pain and/or headache, nasal mucus or stuffiness, cough, and sore throat. What we may not know is that a common herb, found in most kitchens, garlic, is antimicrobial, antifungal, and suitable for a wide range of infectious conditions. Another herb, boneset, promotes sweating and reduces fever, and is also an effective expectorant. This herb is beneficial for feverish colds and flu with muscle pain. Cat-lovers suffering cold misery can use catnip to cool fevers, promote sweating, and help clear mucous congestion.

Back Pain—Alfalfa, Comfrey, Horsetail, Oatstraw, and Slippery Elm

Baldness—Aloe Vera, Horsetail, Jojoba, Kelp, and Oatstraw

Body Odor—Chlorophyll

Bronchitis—Elecampane, Nettle, White Horehound, Cowslip, Thyme

Bruises—Black Walnut, Comfrey, Dandelion, Horsetail, Kelp, Rose Hips, Slippery Elm, White Oak, and Yellow Dock

Burns—Aloe Vera, Comfrey, Horsetail, and Slippery Elm

Cancer—Alfalfa, Astragalus, Burdock Root, Chaparral, Echinacea, Garlic, Onion, Ginko Biloba, Ginseng, Goldenseal, Turmeric

Cholesterol Reduction—Angelica, Black Cohosh, Hawthorn, Hawthorn and Walnut (combination), and Mistletoe

Cold Sores—Aloe Vera, Capsicum (Cayenne), Comfrey, Garlic, Goldenseal, White Oak Bark, and Myrrh (in topical alcohol solution)

Common Cold—Alfalfa or Peppermint (teas), Raspberry (tea), Aloe Vera (drink), Echinacea, Fenugreek, Garlic, Ginger (settles stomach), Goldenseal, Kelp, Marshmallow, Rose Hips, and Slippery Elm (for coughs and throat)

Constipation—Cascara Sagrada, Comfrey, Garlic, Psyllium, Slippery Elm, and Triphala

Dandruff—Burdock and Yucca

Diabetes—Alfalfa, Burdock, Garlic, Goldenseal, Red Clover, Uva Ursi, Watercress, and Yellow Dock

Diarrhea—Alfalfa, Glucomannan, Raspberry (tea), and Slippery Elm

Dieting and Obesity—Bladderwrack (Fucus), Kelp, Garlic, Glucomannan, and Ma Huang

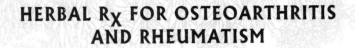

HERBAL Rx FOR OSTEOARTHRITIS AND RHEUMATISM

There are two main types of arthritis. Osteoarthritis (OA) is characterized by pain and swelling of the joints, generally due to wear and tear. Rheumatoid arthritis (RA) is characterized by the inflammation of many joints and requires professional treatment. Rheumatism is a general term for any muscle pain; lumbago is lower-back pain. Symptoms often worsen in damp weather. These are the key systems:

- Stiffness and joint pain
- Swollen or deformed joints
- Hot or burning sensations in joints (RA)
- Creaking sounds in joints

And here are some herbal remedies:

- Angelica is a warming and stimulating herb effective for "cold" types of osteoarthritis and for rheumatism.
- Devil's claw has a potent anti-inflammatory action that has been compared to cortisone. It's better for osteoarthritis and degenerative conditions than for rheumatoid arthritis.
- Bogbean is a cleansing, cooling, and anti-inflammatory herb useful for "hotter" types of arthritis and for muscle pain.
- White willow is rich in salicylates—anti-inflammatories that cool hot joints; it's especially useful for the pain associated with the acute phases of arthritis and for muscle pains.

CHILDHOOD INFECTIONS AND FEVERS

Characterized by sudden swings in body temperature to abnormally high levels, fevers are common in childhood illnesses, and cooling fever herbs can help. Herbs can be used as alternatives to prescribed antibiotics to relieve specific symptoms of mumps, measles, chicken pox, and other infections. For example, purple coneflower contains in its root antibacterial and antiviral properties. It can also strengthen resistance to infection and it is useful for all septic, or infectious conditions. And hyssop is a herb with a relaxing expectorant, especially suitable for children's coughs and respiratory infections.

Research is still in its infancy, especially in the United States, but what is known raises the exciting possibility of being able to predict with reasonable certainty the action a plant chemical will have on humans.

Digestive Disorders—Angelica, Anise, Chamomile, Comfrey, Calamus Root (tea), Dandelion, Fennel, Garlic, Ginger Root, Goldenseal, Papaya or Aloe Vera (with meals), Peppermint, and Slippery Elm

Dry Skin—Alfalfa and Aloe Vera

Energy—Fo-Ti, Ginseng, Gotu Kola

Fatigue—Capsicum (Cayenne), Ginseng, American Ginseng and Red Deer Antler (combination), Gotu Kola, and Oats

Flatulence—Alfalfa, Anise, Blessed Thistle, Capsicum, (Cayenne), Caraway, Fennel, Garlic, Goldenseal, Peppermint, and Wild Yam

Flu—Garlic and Symfre

Foot Odor—Powdered Hemlock Spruce, Powdered Black Walnut Leaf

Gallstones—Chamomile, Dandelion, and Yellow Dock

Gout—Burdock Root, Colchicum (tincture), Guggula, Celery, and White Bryony (tincture—for pain)

Gray Hair—Mulberry Fruit, Privet, Eclipta, Yin Tonics (in general)

Gum Disease—Capsicum (Cayenne), Coneflower, Goldenseal, and Myrrh

Hair Care—Burdock, Chamomile, Comfrey, Horsetail, Jojoba, Nettle, Oat Straw, Peach, Sage, Gotu Kola with Eclipta (together promote hair growth), and Rosemary (helps prevent hair loss)

Headache—Chamomile, Feverfew, Hops, Peppermint plus Catnip (tea for headaches of stomach origin), Red Sage, Skullcap, Spearmint (tea), White Willow, and Wood Betony

Heartburn—Aloe Vera, Burnet, Gentian, and Peppermint

Hemrrhoids—Stone Root (capsule and suppository), and Goldenseal (suppository)

Hepatitis—Celandine (tincture: 1 to 10 drops
three to four times daily), Culver's Root (tincture: 10 to 60 drops three to four times daily),
Fringe Tree (tincture: 5 to 30 drops three to
four times daily), Gymnema Sylvestre, and
Oregon Grape Root

Hives—Alfalfa, Caltrop, Chamomile, Echinacea,
Ginseng, Licorice, Sarsparilla, and Yellow Dock

Hypertension—Ceyenne (Capsicum), Garlic,
Glucomannan, Hawthorn Berries, Hibiscus
Flowers, Hops, Lady's Slipper, Passionflower,
Skullcap, and Valerian

Hypoglycemia—Alfalfa, Aloe Vera (juice), Dandelion, Hawthorn,
Juniper, Kelp, Licorice, Safflower, and Saffron

Immune Deficiency—Alfalfa, Chaparral, Echinacea, Garlic, and
Pau D'Arco

Indigestion—Anise, Fennel, Peppermint and Spearmint

Insect Bites—Aloe Vera (gel), Comfrey, Feverfew, and Papay (for
insect bites); Tea Tree Oil and Goldenseal (as insect repellents)

Insomnia—Catnip, Chamomile, Hops, Lady's Slipper, Skullcap, and
Valerian Root

Itching—Yarrow

Memory—Astragalus, Calamus, Cayenne, Dong Quai, Ginkgo Biloba
Leaf Extract, Ginger, Ginseng, Gotu Kola, and Red Deer Antler

Mental Health—Cayenne, Ginseng, Gotu Kola

Morning Sickness—Alfalfa, Catnip (tea), False Unicorn Root,
Fennel, Ginger Root (capsules or tea), Goldenseal, Kelp, Peppermint
(tea), and Red Raspberry (tea)

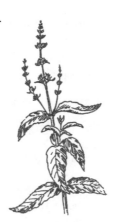

Spearmint

IRON DEFICIENCY

Low hemoglobin levels, which
can be due to a poor diet,
heavy menstruation, or digestive disorders, can lead to a
deficiency of iron in the blood,
which in turn can cause
anemia. Symptoms are breath-
lessness and/or palpitations,
very pale nails or inner eyelids,
or rheumatic-type pains.
Herbal remedies for this condition include dang gui, which
nourishes the blood and invig-
orates the circulation. Another
remedy is stinging nettle, rich
in iron and other minerals.

YELLOW DOCK

An astringent and blood purifier, yellow dock is especially
useful in treating chronic skin
ailments. It is considered one of
the herb kingdom's best blood
builders. By stimulating elimination and improving bile flow, it
nourishes the spleen and liver,
which makes it particularly
useful in treating skin eruptions.

BUTCHER'S BROOM

Varicose veins often are a problem for women. Studies have shown that butcher's broom extract can constrict blood vessels. It contains steroidlike compounds that experts believe can inhibit inflammation and shrink swollen varicose veins. This herb is available in various forms for both internal and external use.

Motion Sickness—Alfalfa, Catnip (tea), False Unicorn Root, Fennel, Ginger Root (capsules or tea), Goldenseal, Kelp, Peppermint (tea), and Red Raspberry (tea)

Nail Problems—Horsetail

Nasal Congestion—Comfrey, Coneflower (*Echinacea angustifolium*), Eucalyptus, Fenugreek, and Magnolia Blossoms (tea)

Nervousness—Betony, Catnip, Chamomile, European Vervain, Hops, Lady's Slipper, Mistletoe, Passionflower, Pulsatilla, Red Sage (for nervous headache), Skullcap, and Valerian

Night Blindness—Bilberry

Osteoporosis—Comfrey and Horsetail

Pain—Black Cohosh Root, Bugleweed, Catnip, Chaparral, Comfrey, Cornsilk, Fenugreek, Hops, Lady's Slipper, Mullein, Pau D'Arco, Valerian, White Willow Bark, Wild Yam (muscle pain), and Wintergreen

Prostate Trouble—Cayenne (Capsicum), False Unicorn Root, Goldenseal, Juniper Berries, Saw Palmetto Berries (oil extract), Siberian Ginseng, and Uva Ursi

Psoriasis—Burdock Root, Chickweed, Common Figwort, Mullein, Slippery Elm (tea), and Yellow American Saffron (tea)

Scurvy—Rose Hips

Skin Problems—Alfalfa, Aloe Vera, Burdock, Comfrey, Dandelion, Goldenseal, Horsetail, Oatstraw, Queen of the Meadow, Yarrow, Yellow Dock

Smoking—Hops, Skullcap, Valerian, Catnip, Slippery Elm

Stress—Alfalfa, Chamomile, Ginseng, Gotu Kola, Hops, Kelp, Lady's Slipper, Passionflower, and Valerian

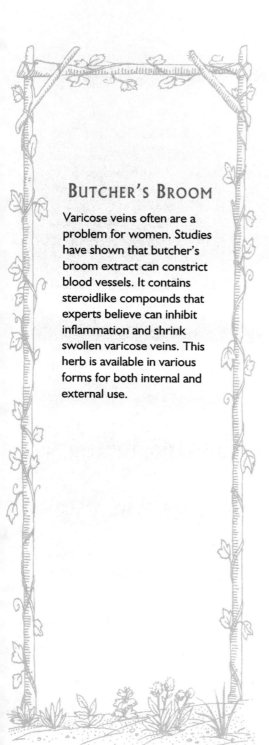

Valerian

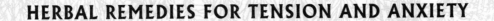

HERBAL REMEDIES FOR TENSION AND ANXIETY

Excessive stress can lead to a variety of health problems that are not obviously linked to tension. Stress can also complicate pre-existing conditions. These are the key symptoms:

- Inability to relax
- Emotional instability/mood swings
- Headaches
- Sleeplessness

Here are some herbal remedies:

- Linden reduces nervous tension and helps prevent arteriosclerosis.
- Pasque flower contains nervine and anodyne with sedative action. It is useful for nervous and sexual problems.
- Skullcap acts as a relaxant and restorative for the central nervous system. It is good for nervous debility.
- Wood betony is a sedative that acts to calm the nervous system by soothing fearfulness and invigorating exhaustion.
- Vervain is a relaxing nervine with a tonic effect on the liver.

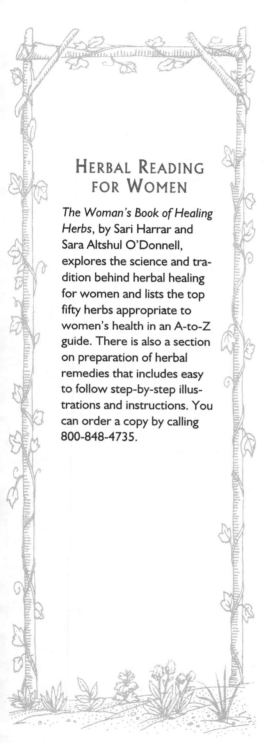

HERBAL READING FOR WOMEN

The Woman's Book of Healing Herbs, by Sari Harrar and Sara Altshul O'Donnell, explores the science and tradition behind herbal healing for women and lists the top fifty herbs appropriate to women's health in an A-to-Z guide. There is also a section on preparation of herbal remedies that includes easy to follow step-by-step illustrations and instructions. You can order a copy by calling 800-848-4735.

Tonsillitis and Sore Throat—Echinacea, Bayberry Root, Ginger Root, Goldenseal (gargle), Marigold Flowers (tincture as throat swab), Pleurisy Root, and St. John's wort

Tooth Decay—Horsetail, and Peppermint Oil (toothaches)

Urinary Tract Infections—Barberry (Uva Ursi) (tincture), Buchu, Couch Grass (tincture), Echinacea, Garlic, Goldenseal (tea), Juniper Berries, Parsley Root and Seed (tea or tincture)

Varicose Veins—Butcher's Broom, Capiscum, Goldenseal, Horsetail, Kelp Oatstraw, Parsley, White Oak Bark, Witch Hazel

Warts—Aloe Vera, Black Walnut (externally), Garlic, Goldenseal, and Tea Tree Oil (externally)

Worms—Black Walnut, Blessed Thistle, Cranberry (concentrate), Garlic, Grapefruit Seed Extract, Pink Root, Senna, and Slippery Elm

Yeast Infections—Echinacea, Garlic

For Women Especially

The natural functions of women are not technically "ailments" or "illnesses," and, therefore, were not covered in the preceding list of common ailments. However, these natural functions can be uncomfortable or painful or even life threatening.

There are a number of herbs that can help the female body deal with the hormonal changes brought on by the menopausal phase in a woman's life. These include chasteberry, motherwort, St. John's wort, and (for vaginal dryness, hot flashes, and mood swings) black cohosh.

Black cohosh should be a standardized extract of which 40 to 80 milligrams should be taken twice daily, depending on the severity of the symptoms. Often, black cohosh will be completely effective on its own, but it is always important to remember that every woman is an individual, and every woman's body, psychology, mental attitude, and other attributes of her personality are different. What may work for one may not work for another. (A naturopathic physician can blend a special botanical formula based on each woman's particular needs.)

As a woman, you already know your own body better than any health care practitioner, and you need to be able to rely on your own experience of your feminine bodily functions to act as a guide when using herbal remedies to aid your natural processes.

It is important to bear in mind that menopause is a natural progression in every woman's life not a sickness to be treated or cured. And since every woman has a different response to this natural process affecting her body, her emotions, and often her entire life, it is necessary for each individual to look for the approach that works best for her.

In addition, there are natural forms of the hormones progesterone and estrogen that can be used to supplement herbal remedies. Many women react well to these natural hormones, which are available in capsules and creams.

Researchers have discovered that some foods have a high level of phytoestrogens, or soy isoflavones. These are not true hormones. They are a 100 percent natural product made from plants that seem to have the ability to balance the decline in natural hormonal activity that occurs during menopause. Women interested in further information on these and other herbs can visit the American Botanical Council's Web site at *www.herbalgram.org*.

Herbs to Avoid During Pregnancy and While Lactating

Agave and **Yucca** contain large quantities of irritating saponins.

Aloe is a purgative.

Autumn Crocus (otherwise known as SAFFRON). In large doses, it can cause miscarriage.

Bearberry bark contains similar alkaloids to goldenseal; berries and leaves are alright.

Birthroot contains oxytocin.

Black Cohosh can irritate the uterus.

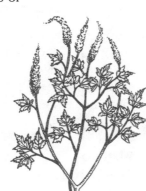
Black Cohosh

NATUROPATHIC PHYSICIANS

For referrals, contact the following associations:

American Association of Naturopathic Physicians
2366 Eastlake Avenue, Suite 322
Seattle, Washington 98102.
206-298-0125
Web site:
www.naturopathic.org

Or contact one of two U.S. Department of Education accredited naturopathic colleges:

Bastyr University
144 NE 54th Street
Seattle, Washington 98105
206-523-9585
Web site:
www.bastyr.edu/alumni/

National College of Naturopathic Medicine
049 SW Porter
Portland, Oregon 97201
Web site:
www.ncnm.edu/sap.htm

NONHERBAL HOME-BASED MEDICAL SUPPLIES

In addition to the herbs and herbal preparations in your first-aid department, you should include other items basic to the delivery of home-based medical treatments, such as sharp scissors, a variety of bandages and tape, sterile absorbent gauze pads, tweezers, and elastic bandages (for sprains), as well as rubbing alcohol and hydrogen peroxide for disinfecting wounds and abrasions before applying a herbal remedy and/or bandaging.

You should also keep some nonherbal products on hand, such as baking soda, which can be made with water into a healing paste for burns and insect stings, and cider vinegar, which will soothe rashes caused by contact with poison ivy, poison oak, and poison sumac.

Blue Cohosh contains oxytocin.

Buckthorn is a purgative.

Cascara Sagrada is a purgative.

Comfrey contains alkaloids in the roots that are dangerous to the liver; the leaves are safe.

Cotton Root Bark contains oxytocin.

Dong Quai contains coumarins that can irritate the uterus and liver.

Feverfew

Ephedra or **Ma Huang** increases blood pressure and can cause irregular heartbeat, insomnia, and headaches.

Evening Primrose Oil induces labor.

Feverfew contains essential oils that can damage liver and kidneys.

Flax Seeds in large doses may stimulate uterine contractions.

Goldenseal contains irritating alkaloids that stress the liver and kidneys.

Juniper Berries are very harsh on the kidneys.

Licorice increases blood pressure; in large doses it can cause heart failure, headache, lethargy, water retention, and excessive excretion of potassium.

Mints such as basil, catnip, rosemary, thyme, savory, peppermint, oregano, ground ivy, sage, and spearmint contain essential oils that (used internally—or extracted into a tincture), may harm the kidneys and liver; the infusion, taken in large enough quantity, may stimulate uterine contractions.

Mistletoe in large doses can damage the heart.

Mistletoe (American) can raise blood pressure and cause uterine contractions.

Mugwort/Cronewort can be used to help induce labor.

Nutmeg contains essential oils that can adversely affect the brain, liver, and kidneys when taken in large doses.

Osha can irritate the uterus.

Parsley is a well-known and very effective abortifacient.

Pennyroyal contains essential oils that can harm kidneys and liver and can cause miscarriage.

Poke Root in large doses (more than four drops) may stress the kidneys.

Rue contains essential oils that can damage kidneys and liver.

Senna is a potent purgative.

Southernwood contains essential oils, similar to those in wormwood, that are easily extracted into tinctures and that can cause brain damage.

Tansy contains essential oils in tinctures that can damage kidneys and liver.

Thuja contains essential oils that can damage the kidneys and liver.

Turkey Rhubarb is a purgative; it can cause uterine contractions.

Wormwood contains essential oils that can cause brain damage.

Herbal First Aid

Whether you grow your own herbs and make your own herbal preparations or use those that are grown and prepared commercially using modern methods, it's a good idea to have an "herbal first aid kit" on hand at all times. Many commercially available herbal preparations—capsules, tablets, bulk herbs, tinctures, extracts—offer valuable healing properties, so it only makes sense to keep a supply of these in your home medicine cabinet. This is especially applicable to preparations that are useful for first aid, when you need

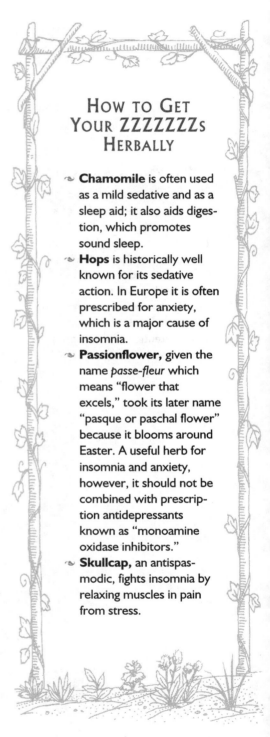

HOW TO GET YOUR ZZZZZZZs HERBALLY

- **Chamomile** is often used as a mild sedative and as a sleep aid; it also aids digestion, which promotes sound sleep.
- **Hops** is historically well known for its sedative action. In Europe it is often prescribed for anxiety, which is a major cause of insomnia.
- **Passionflower,** given the name *passe-fleur* which means "flower that excels," took its later name "pasque or paschal flower" because it blooms around Easter. A useful herb for insomnia and anxiety, however, it should not be combined with prescription antidepressants known as "monoamine oxidase inhibitors."
- **Skullcap,** an antispasmodic, fights insomnia by relaxing muscles in pain from stress.

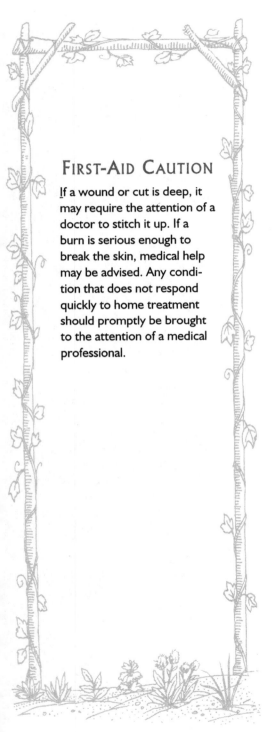

First-Aid Caution

If a wound or cut is deep, it may require the attention of a doctor to stitch it up. If a burn is serious enough to break the skin, medical help may be advised. Any condition that does not respond quickly to home treatment should promptly be brought to the attention of a medical professional.

instant access to remedies that can stave off infection or other problems until you can get to your health care practitioner.

Herbal remedies can be used for quick and effective relief over a wide range of everyday mishaps that occur around the home—from the stings of insects such as wasps and bees to minor burns, scrapes, cuts, and sprained ankles.

The section that follows provides a list of those herbs that are of the most value for treating minor wounds (abrasions, cuts, and burns) such as marigold, witch hazel, and arnica, as well as those that have antiseptic properties and are extremely valuable for their anti-infection qualities—such as clove oil, eucalyptus oil, and lavender oil.

We also include the Bach Rescue Remedy—a combination of flower remedies (find out more about flower remedies in Chapter 8)—for use in emergency situations that involve shock—physical or emotional upset from experiences such as a fall or the receiving of bad news.

We also include those herbs to keep on hand to treat common ailments—colds, flu, upset stomach—such as echinacea, fenugreek, garlic, and ginger. It is always best to treat any incipient illness promptly to prevent it from taking hold of one's system.

Study the list of herbs and their uses and decide which are most appropriate for you and your family. Chamomile, for example, is excellent for relaxation; if you or members of your family suffer from stress, you might decide to keep a good supply of this useful herb. Or, if you or any of your family members suffer from occasional insomnia, you may decide to keep a supply of lemon balm available. (It should be noted that persistent or chronic insomnia may require the assistance of a professional.)

Herbal First Aid Kit

Aloe Vera Gel is known for its effectiveness for burns and rashes, it can also be used for insect bites and stings, poison oak and ivy, acne, and itch.

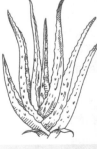

Aloe Vera

Antispasmodic Extract is made of valerian, anise, lobelia, black walnut, brigham tea, licorice, and ginger. It soothes nerves and spastic conditions, is excellent in emergencies (e.g., to calm hysteria or shock brought on by poisonous bites/stings), and can be used externally for pain and muscular spasms.

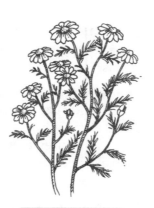

Chamomile

Arnica is useful for sprains and bruises.

Bilberry contains antioxidants known to help maintain capillary strength. Bilberry is known as the herbal sight saver because many vision problems are the result of minute ruptures of capillaries in the eyes. Drink bilberry tea to strengthen your vision.

Capsicum powder and extract can be rubbed on toothaches, inflammation, and swellings. In treating arthritis, rub capsicum extract over the inflamed joint and wrap with flannel overnight. It is also useful to stop internal and external bleeding by helping to normalize circulation. Capsicum and plantain will draw out foreign bodies embedded in the skin.

Cascara Sagrada is a safe tonic and laxative; keeps bowels open in illness and prevents constipation.

Chamomile, used as a tea, is safe for treating children's colds, indigestion, and nervous disorders. It relieves menstrual cramps and is relaxing as a treatment for insomnia. Chamomile can also be applied to swellings, sore muscles, and painful joints. It also contains an oil that relaxes the smooth muscles in the stomach. Brew a tea with 1 or 2 teaspoons of leaves in 1 cup of boiling water.

Charcoal is often used in the treatment of diarrhea and intestinal gas. It can also be used to treat some poisonings, or as a poultice.

Chlorophyll (liquid) is a good cleanser for the blood and the bowels. Rich in minerals, it is nutritious for children and nursing mothers.

MONEY IS NOT THE ISSUE

Proof that today's consumers take alternative medicine very seriously is shown by the statistics: Americans make approximately 630 million visits to alternative practitioners every year, in comparison with only 385 million visits to primary care physicians. In 1997, they spent $12 billion out of their own pockets for alternative treatments not covered by standardized medical insurance.

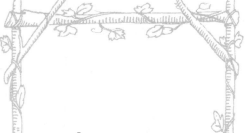

INFORMATION ON-LINE

For up-to-date information about the latest in natural healing, check out *Prevention* on-line at *www.healthyideas.com* Look for other Web sites, too, as more are coming on-line.

BLOOD PRESSURE CAUTION

People taking medication to lower their blood pressure should avoid licorice (the herb, not the candy), mistletoe, and eleuthero, according to Varro E. Tyler, Ph.D, Sc.D., advisor to *Prevention* magazine. Tyler also warns those using thyroid medication to avoid bugleweed, which can further decrease thyroid activity.

Clove Oil soothes the pain of a toothache. Due to its antiseptic properties, it is also useful in the treatment of cuts.

Comfrey as an ointment or infusion helps to heal bruises and cuts. It encourages the growth of scar tissue. Comfrey, when made into a strong decoction, can also be used to stop bleeding. It can be used internally and externally for the healing of fractures, wounds, sores, and ulcers.

Composition Essence, including elderflower and peppermint, is a good remedy for colds and flu.

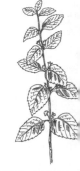

Lemon Balm

Echinacea, the body's defensive line, activates virus-fighting blood cells and stops a cold virus from spreading. It comes in capsule and tincture form.

Eucalyptus Oil is good for bronchial spasms, chills, colds, sore throat, and rheumatism, and functions as an expectorant. It is also used in aromatherapy and herbalism to treat cuts and boils.

Fenugreek helps dissolve mucus in sinus infections and bronchitis. This herb also lowers fever temperature and is excellent for children.

Feverfew relieves headaches by constricting blood flow and reducing inflammation. Take 125 milligrams daily for pain relief.

Flowers and **Plants**, edible and nutritious, include Chicory, Clover, Dandelion, Elderberry, Squash, Borage, Nasturtium, Lamb's Quarters, Plaintain, Purslane, Rose Petals, Violets, and Wild Watercress.

Garlic fights heart disease by inhibiting the production of cholesterol. Garlic oil, "nature's antibiotic," is used for earaches. Taking garlic with capsicum and vitamin C at the beginning of a cold is often effective.

Ginger soothes upset stomachs, nausea, colds, and flu.

Lavender Oil is well known for its antiseptic, antibacterial, and wound-healing properties. It is also very important in aromatherapy.

HELPFUL HERBS FOR THE URINARY TRACT

COMMON NAME	SCIENTIFIC NAME	ACTION
Bearberry (leaves)	*Arctostaphylos uva ursi*	Antiseptic
Birch (leaves)	*Betula spp.*	Aquaretic
Goldenrod (leaves and tops)	*Solidago spp.*	Aquaretic
Lovage (root)	*Levisticum officinale*	Aquaretic
Parsley	*Petroselinum crispum*	Aquaretic

Lemon Balm is a good herb for children's stomach upsets and situations in which a relaxing effect is needed.

Licorice is an ancient cough remedy. It generates a productive cough and speeds recovery. It comes in lozenge form or as a tea.

Lobelia Extract relaxes spasms, internally and externally. A few drops in the ear relieve earaches. Mixing lobelia with catnip as an enema is effective for fevers and infections.

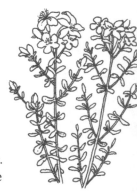

St. John's Wort

Marigold is one of the most effective remedies for cuts and cold sores.

Peppermint Oil soothes nausea, assists in digestion, cleanses and tones the body, relaxes the body, and quiets the restless.

Red Raspberry is excellent during pregnancy; it relieves nausea, prevents hemorrhage, reduces pain, and eases childbirth. It is also reliable for children's stomachaches, fevers, colds, and flu.

Sarsaparilla made into a hot decoction with an ounce of root in a pint of water will promote profuse sweating and act as a powerful agent to expel gas from the stomach and intestines.

Slippery Elm is good for digestion. Use slippery elm powder to help bring boils to a head.

St. John's Wort, "the herbal antidepressant," is popular for the treatment of depression and mood disorders. As an oil, it is a useful remedy for burns and minor wounds.

Tea Tree Oil has antifungal properties, which are helpful with conditions such as athlete's foot, acne, boils, burns, warts, vaginal infections, tonsillitis, sinus infections, ringworm, skin rashes, impetigo, herpes, corns, head lice, cold sores, canker sores, insect bites, and other fungal infections.

Witch Hazel is widely used for its astringent and blood-clotting actions, witch hazel is one of the most widely used first-aid remedies. It can be used as a compress for minor burns and sprains or applied directly to insect bites, nosebleeds, and cuts.

Medicine of the People

Herbalism has always been considered the "medicine of the people," consisting of simple remedies (in medieval times herbs were called "simples") to be used at home to treat minor ailments or wounds. Herbs have also been used as a supplement to prescription drugs given for chronic and acute conditions. Many herbs can be easily prepared as teas, and more complex preparations can be made at home (see Chapter 11). Most people choose commercially prepared herbal products available at health food stores and some pharmacies. It is important to keep in mind that although most herbs are considered to be safe, they can be potent and should be treated respectfully. Never exceed the recommended doses, and do not continue with home treatment if a condition worsens or becomes chronic. If the true diagnosis is in any way uncertain, a professional should be consulted.

Although some herbs work quickly, especially for acute conditions, chronic problems may require several weeks, or even months, of treatment before significant results are achieved. With herbal treatments, symptoms may change as time progresses, so it is necessary to review the remedy and its effects periodically—at least once a month—and to be prepared to alter it in accord with changing conditions. Professional herbalists, who monitor their patients, often adjust their remedies frequently as the person's general state changes. Self-reliance and self-treatment are admirable, but due caution must always be taken, especially if the person is taking any prescription medicines for a particular condition. Some herbs interact with prescription drugs; therefore, you should *always* consult your doctor or health care professional before using herbal remedies in conjunction with prescription medicines.

TEENAGER'S TERROR

The inflammation of the sebaceous glands in the skin, known as acne, is the teenager's scourge. These are the key symptoms:

- Inflamed pustules
- Excessively oily skin
- Infected cysts and scarring in severe cases

Effective herbs include the following:

- Garlic contains antibacterial and antifungal properties. It provides good antiseptic action for infected skin conditions.
- Cabbage contains both antibacterial and anti-inflammatory properties. It is nutritive and healing.
- Tea Tree Oil is a potent antibacterial agent for infected skin.

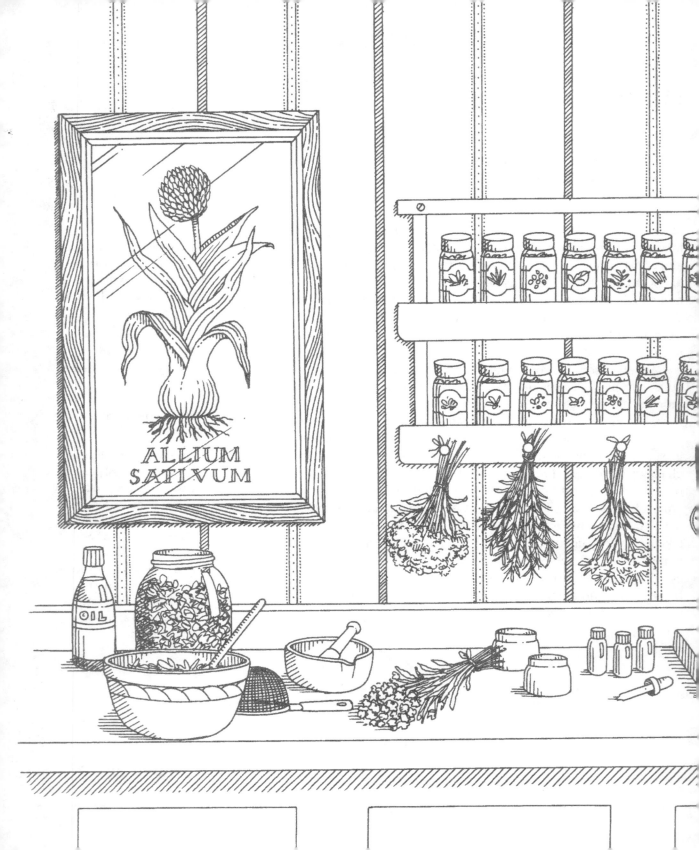

ALLIUM
SATIVUM

OIL

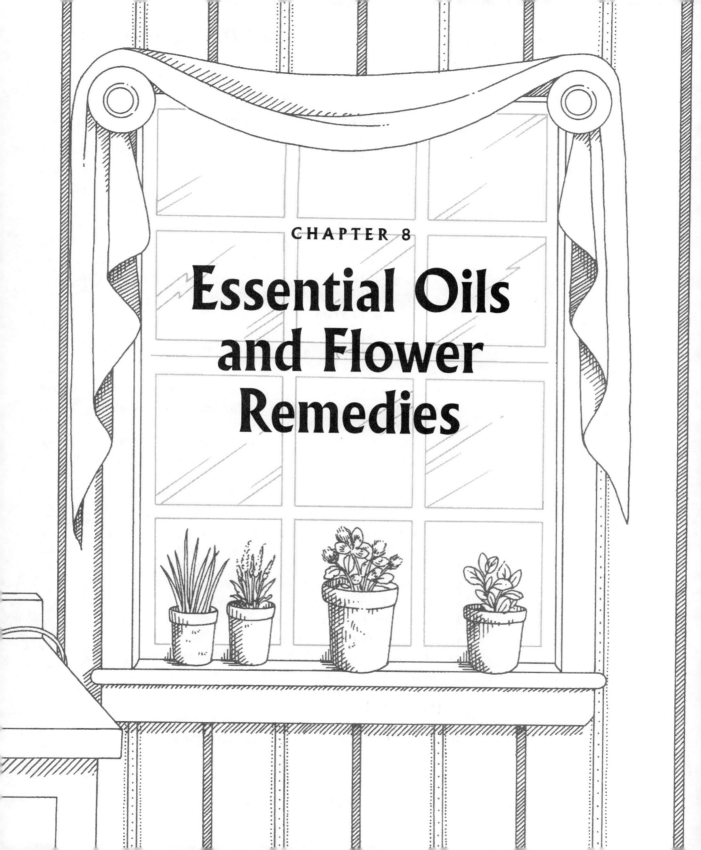

CHAPTER 8

Essential Oils and Flower Remedies

A History of Essential Oils

Essential oils are one of the great untapped resources of the world. The concentrated essences of various flowers, fruits, herbs, and plants have been used for centuries all over the world, but in modern times we have forgotten the power of these ancient medicines of the earth, preferring instead to use the products of perfume and chemical companies which imitate the natural fragrances and medicinal and cleansing properties of essential oils. Because the essential oils are so sweet-smelling, many people suppose their value is essentially one of charm and fragrance—but this is a mistake. Modern scientific research has proven that essential oils are potent, with remarkable medicinal properties.

—VALERIE ANN WORWOOD, *The Complete Book of Essential Oils & Aromatherapy*

How, one might wonder, is it possible to extract those tiny droplets we call "essential oils" from the bulk of the plant material? And how can these extracted oils be stored?

Given that this secret was known some 5000 years ago in Egypt, it seems quite odd that it has been so often "lost" through the ages and has had to be constantly rediscovered.

Archaeologists discovered distillation devices in Mesopotamia, c. 5000 B.C.E., and Egypt was using essential oils as early as 4000 B.C.E. The most frequently used oils in that ancient era were distilled from cedar, cinnamon, lily, turpentine, dill, basil, and coriander—all plants still familiar to us today. Used for healing as well as cosmetic purposes—and for ritual ceremonies—essential oils were known in Babylon, India, and China. After their conquest of the Egyptian Empire, the Romans incorporated the knowledge of essential oils into their culture.

However, there are no records suggesting that essential oils were used after the fall of the Roman

Empire. They reappeared at the end of the 10th century in Arab countries where physicians used them to treat patients. It is believed that the famous Arabian physician who went by his European name of Avicenna (980–1037) rediscovered the method for extracting the precious oils from plants. Later, after their conquest of Spain, the Moors taught the art of extracting essential oils at universities that they founded in Spain. However, with the ouster of the Arabs from Spain, essential oils once again fell into disuse.

Ironically, the first major indication of the antiseptic properties of essential oils in Europe came from the fact that perfumers—who handled the oils daily as part of their profession—were seemingly immune to the plague known as the "Black Death" and to the epidemics of cholera that periodically swept Europe during the Middle Ages. By the late 17th century, the oils were back in use, primarily as medicinals. Toward the end of the 19th century, scientific experiments into the antibacterial properties of plants began to clarify the chemical composition and potential healing powers of essential oils. Alas, and as usual, instead of this discovery leading to an increase in the use of essential oils, scientists attempted to mimic their properties in order to create synthetic chemical substitutes.

It was the work of a French chemist, René-Maurice Gattefossé, in the early 1900s that brought renewed interest to this form of healing. Considered the "father of modern aromatherapy," Dr. Gattefossé coined the term *aromatherapy* when he used it as the title of a book he published in 1937. He was especially interested in the medicinal aspects of essential oils.

During World War II, another French physician, Dr. Jean Valnet, who had been much impressed with Gattefossé's findings, used essential oils in the treatment of wounds received by soldiers in wartime Europe. He used the oils to disinfect and heal and, in turn, published a book, *Aromathérapie, Traitement des maladies par les essences des plantes.*

Fortunately, Dr. Valnet was interested in teaching other physicians the medical uses of essential oils, and as a result, there are today more than a thousand physicians in France who use essential oils in their practices.

During the 1920s, Italian scientists conducted experiments with the psychological effects of essential oils. Two of them, Dr. Renato

SCENTS AND SENSIBILITY

Essential oils affect people through the sense of smell, which is the most potent of all the senses because the information is delivered straight to the hypothalymus. As moods, motivation, and creativity all stem from the hypothalymus, odors affect all of these processes. Think of a disgusting odor and how it can affect your appetite—or think of a fragrance that brings back a pleasant memory of a loved one, and you'll get the idea of how intimately intertwined scents are with our emotions, memories, and ideas.

Cayola and Dr. Giovanni Garri, published an article in 1922 discussing the effects of essential oils on the nervous system. They had not only observed the bacteria-destroying capacities of the oil, but they had studied their stimulating and calming effects, as well.

Another Italian, Professor Paolo Rovesti, at the University of Milan, conducted research on the psychological effects of essential oils, treating patients afflicted with depression and hysteria. He recommended a variety of combinations of the oils. For example, for depression, he recommended combining jasmine, sandalwood, orange blossom, verbena, and lemon oil.

How Essential Oils Work

Today, people all over the world are paying attention to the healing effects of essential oils, and scientists are continuing to conduct research in an attempt to understand more about the effects of these amazing aromas on the human mind, body, and psychology.

Essential oils are extracted from the aromatic essences of certain plants, trees, fruit, flowers, herbs, and spices. Natural volatile oils, they have identifiable chemical and medicinal properties. At this point, over 150 have been extracted, and each has its own definitive scent and unique healing properties. Oils are produced from a wide range of plants, from the exotic jasmine to the garden-variety parsley. For optimum benefit, the oils must be extracted from natural raw ingredients, with attention to purity. They must be stored in dark, tightly stoppered glass bottles and kept away from light and heat in order to maintain their potency. They can be used individually or in combination.

Despite considerable research, the chemistry of essential oils is not fully understood. Each oil, by current count, contains at least 100 *different* constituents that are chemically classified. And scientists figure there may be many chemical compounds yet to be identified.

Thus, the oils and their actions are extremely complex. In addition to being antiseptic, each also possesses individual properties. The collective qualities of each oil give it a dominant characteristic, whether it be stimulating, calming, energizing, or relaxing. Essential oils have obvious psychological effects, and they also have notable physiological effects, which means that within the

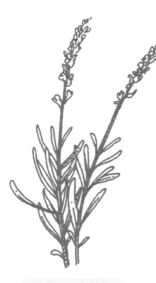

Lavendar

body, they are able to operate in three ways: pharmacologically, physiologically, and psychologically. From the pharmacological perspective, the oils react with body chemistry similarly to drugs, but with a slower and more sympathetic effect and with fewer side effects. In addition, certain oils have a particular affinity for different body parts—spice oils, for example, tend to benefit the digestive system.

Some oils, like lavender, are known as adaptogens, which, as the name implies, adapt to whatever condition needs assistance. The psychological effect is triggered by the connection the aromatic molecules make with the brain.

Although aromatherapy is compatible with herbal remedies and conventional medicine, it should not be used under the following conditions without the consultation of a qualified practitioner:

- If you are pregnant
- If you have allergies
- If you have a chronic medical condition such as high blood pressure or epilepsy
- If you are receiving medical or psychiatric treatment
- If you are taking homeopathic remedies
- If you have any chronic or serious health problem such as a heart condition.

However, aromatherapy is safe to use at home for minor or short-term problems, such as mild depression, tension, or minor ills, so long as you follow safety guidelines.

Anyone wanting to use essential oils can avail themselves of a wealth of additional information for every need quite easily. One good Internet source is *www.geocities.com/~aromaweb/*. This Web site will provide tips for beginners and information about where to buy essential oils and will allow you to look up books and contact experts. The advice here is straightforward and no-nonsense—written by real people who know their stuff, not by manufacturers or someone trying to sell you something. You can also check the resources section in the back of this book for suppliers of herbal products, including essential oils.

OILS TO AVOID

Not all natural plants or essentials oils are beneficial. According to Valerie Ann Worwood in The Complete Book of Essential Oils and Aromatherapy, the following essential oils should never be used.

Bitter almond
Boldo leaf
Calamus
Yellow camphor
Horseradish
Jaborandi leaf
Mugwort
Mustard
Pennyroyal
Rue
Sassafras
Savin
Southernwood
Tansy
Thuja
Wintergreen
Wornseed
Wormwood

Flower Remedies

Emotions can kill you, literally—emotional harmony and balance are the basis of health and well-being. Negative thoughts are as dangerous to your health as are bacteria and viruses. Positive thoughts and feelings can even protect you from becoming infected. And if you do become ill or have an accident, the power of a positive outlook will speed your natural healing process.

Flower essences are prescribed for emotional or psychological conditions or types. They have been called "nature's Prozac." Because they penetrate through subtle vibrational means, as do homeopathic preparations used to treat physical problems, they can be extraordinarily effective over a broad range of conditions. My 10 years of studying and using them for myself and my clients has proved them effective in improving health through restoring emotional balance.

Flower essence remedies are homeopathic preparations one can easily self-prescribe. Numerous books are available on the subject, and complete descriptions of each remedy are available from their sellers, as are tests that can be self-administered to determine which remedies apply to you (see the listing at the end of this chapter).

These essences come in liquid form and are administered diluted in pure water. Extracted from flowers and plants, they are not a drug or a chemical but derive from the traditional idea that plants contain healing properties. In fact, many of our drugs are based on plant derivative or synthetic replicates of them. As stated earlier, the ingredient in aspirin, for example, was originally extracted from the bark of the willow tree.

The theory behind essences is the same as I have already posited: that our inner states effect our physical condition. It is well known, for example, that so-called type A people, with a tough, aggressive, hard-driving style, are at risk for heart disease. Now, however, it is being recognized, according to a study by psychologist Tilmer Engebretson at Ohio State University in Columbus, that people who have a trait he names "cynical hostility" are at greater risk for developing heart-tissue damage than are their

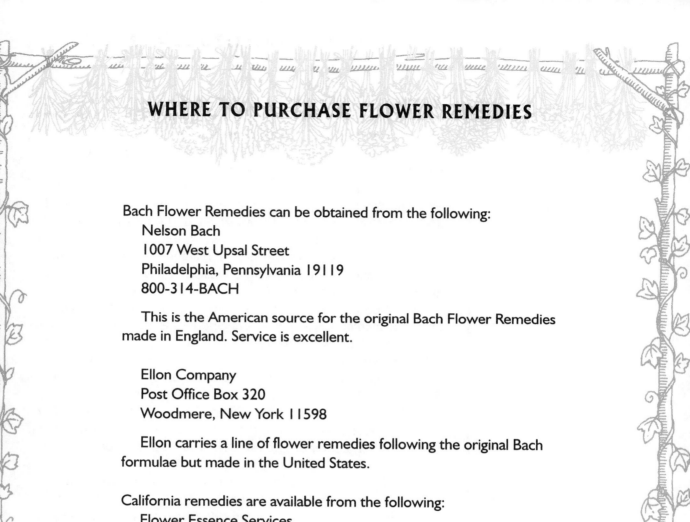

WHERE TO PURCHASE FLOWER REMEDIES

Bach Flower Remedies can be obtained from the following:
Nelson Bach
1007 West Upsal Street
Philadelphia, Pennsylvania 19119
800-314-BACH

This is the American source for the original Bach Flower Remedies made in England. Service is excellent.

Ellon Company
Post Office Box 320
Woodmere, New York 11598

Ellon carries a line of flower remedies following the original Bach formulae but made in the United States.

California remedies are available from the following:
Flower Essence Services
Post Office Box 586
Nevada City, California 94939

Other remedies are available from:
Pegasus Products Inc.
Post Office Box 228
Boulder, Colorado 80306

nonhostile colleagues. Other reports have shown a connection between hostility in healthy people and the subsequent development of atherosclerosis and high cholesterol. One study at Duke University showed that cynicism, mistrust, and aggressive anger increased the death rate from heart disease.

By treating these emotional stress conditions that underlie disease and illness, we get at the root of the problem directly. A real and lasting change in attitude toward self and others is readily observed by those who take the remedies. It may seem odd to you that flower extracts can make such far-reaching changes in a personality, but a study made by Michael Weisglas, Ph.D., for his dissertation, has demonstrated the effectiveness of the essences.

The oldest and longest tested flower essences are the Bach Flower Remedies, developed in England in the 1930s by Dr. Edward Bach, a physician who was dismayed at the lack of success he was achieving with the medical methods of his day. He gave up a successful Harley Street practice in 1930 to devote himself exclusively to finding remedies in the plant world that would enable his suffering patients to overcome the emotional conditions that beset them—fear, worry, depression—and to assist in their own healing. Says Dr. Phillip M. Chancellor, author of *The Handbook of Bach Flower Remedies*:

It is well known that a long continued fear or worry will deplete an individual's vitality; it will cause him to feel out of sorts, below par or not himself. Under these conditions the body loses its natural resistance to disease. It is in a fit state to become the prey of any infection and any form of illness.

The Remedies are still prepared exclusively by the Dr. Edward Bach Healing Center in England. Of them, John Diamond, M.D. has this to say:

There is no doubt of their tremendous efficacy. They are as potent as any therapeutic substances that we have for raising the life energy of the individual. Dr. Bach never meant them to be therapeutic in the sense of primarily curing physical disease, but rather as overcoming the

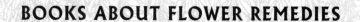

BOOKS ABOUT FLOWER REMEDIES

The Bach Flower Remedies by Edward Bach, M.D., and F. J. Wheeler, M.D., is considered the "bible" on the Bach Flower Remedies. This book is written by the man who developed them.

Handbook of the Bach Flower Remedies by Dr. Phillip M. Chancellor is the book I recommend most for anyone wanting to learn the Bach Flower Remedies. Keyword descriptions of the remedies are followed by complete descriptions of the personality traits to which each is applicable. Numerous case histories detail the remedies used for specific conditions and the physical ailments that were healed as a result.

Flower Remedies Handbook, Emotional Healing and Growth with Bach and Other Flower Essences by Donna Cunningham is a recently published (1992) compendium by an excellent author who is also an astrologer. In 1986, Professional Astrologers Inc. gave her their annual award for her lifetime contributions to the field. This book is highly recommended.

The Flower Essence Journal, Flower Essence Services, Post Office Box 586, Nevada City, California 94939, is a periodical/newsletter covering flower essences and their uses.

mental correlates of physical disease so as to allow the inhibited life energy to manifest itself and to proceed with the healing process, the true healing—that which comes from within.

Here are some examples of flower essences and their uses:

- Vine—for the desire to control and dominate
- Willow—for resentment and bitterness
- Chicory—for possessive martyr types
- Heather—for the lonely and self-absorbed
- White chestnut—for worry and mental obsession.

A special blend of essences used to treat emergency conditions such as shock, physical or emotional, is called Rescue Remedy. I keep a small bottle in my purse. The remedies can be placed directly under the tongue if water is not available. My diabetic cat once went into convulsions, and I saved his life by putting a drop of the Rescue Remedy on his tongue.

Another especially useful remedy is Star of Bethlehem, one of the components of the Rescue Remedy. It is for the *after effect* of shock, mental or physical, and is marvelously effective for anyone who has suffered trauma, especially in childhood. Dr. Bach called this remedy, "the comforter and soother of pains and sorrows." One of his patients wrote:

When I look back, I see that nearly all of my illnesses were the result of shock. Certainly my rheumatoid arthritis was! I was accused of breaking an old and valuable Chinese plate, which I did not do. This was such a shock to me that my hands became stiff, and I had to give up my music.

Shock can go deep into the system and manifest as illness long after the original incident. For example, childhood sexual molestation can cause severe pelvic pain in adult women.

Similar to the Rescue Remedy is the Five-Flower Formula from Healing Herbs English Flower Essences.

The California Flower Essences, developed during the 1970s, reflect their era—they are specific to conditions such as spiritual growth and self-actualization, alienation, and isolation—all New Age concerns. Here are some examples:

- Shooting Star—for feeling alienated
- Dogwood—for receptivity to love
- Mariposa lily—for the feeling of separateness
- Bleeding heart—for releasing painful emotional attachments

The remedies can be used alone or as part of your health maintenance program or for healing purposes. Often when people take the self-test, they mark 10 or 20 remedies that apply to them—an indication of how emotionally stressed many of us are. However, it is best to take no more than four at one time. Think of essences as lifelong friends, changing them as you change, carefully selecting them for your current state. If you use a pendulum, you can use it to check your selections with it. They are not difficult to learn, and they are a comforting companion on your healing journey.

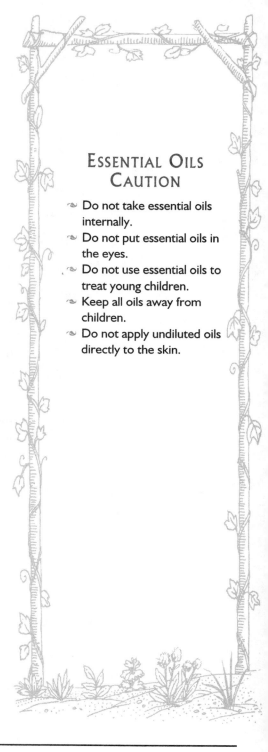

ESSENTIAL OILS CAUTION

- Do not take essential oils internally.
- Do not put essential oils in the eyes.
- Do not use essential oils to treat young children.
- Keep all oils away from children.
- Do not apply undiluted oils directly to the skin.

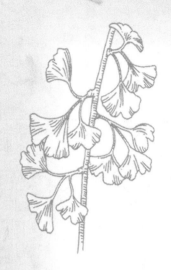

Part Three

HERBAL
HEALING TODAY

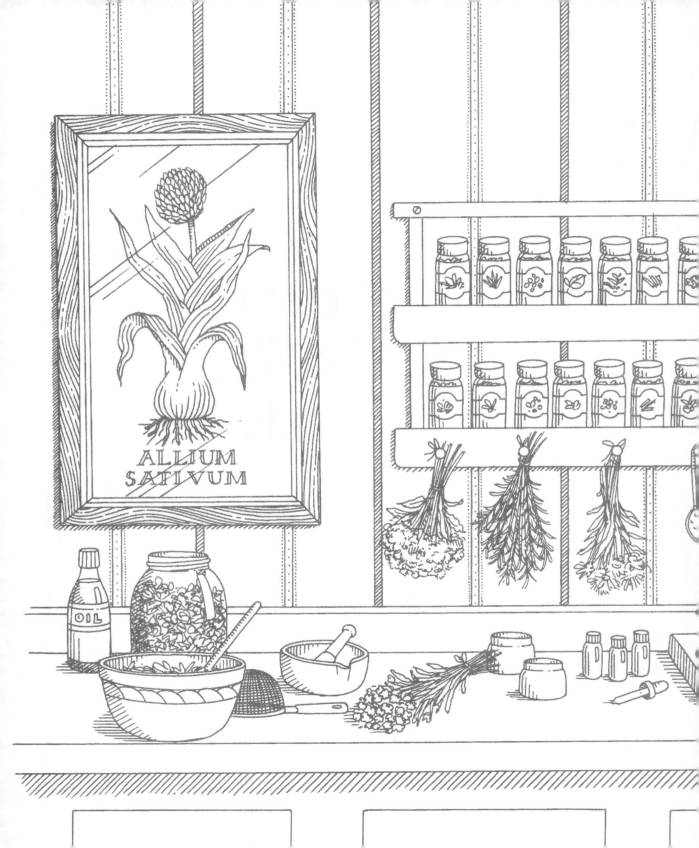

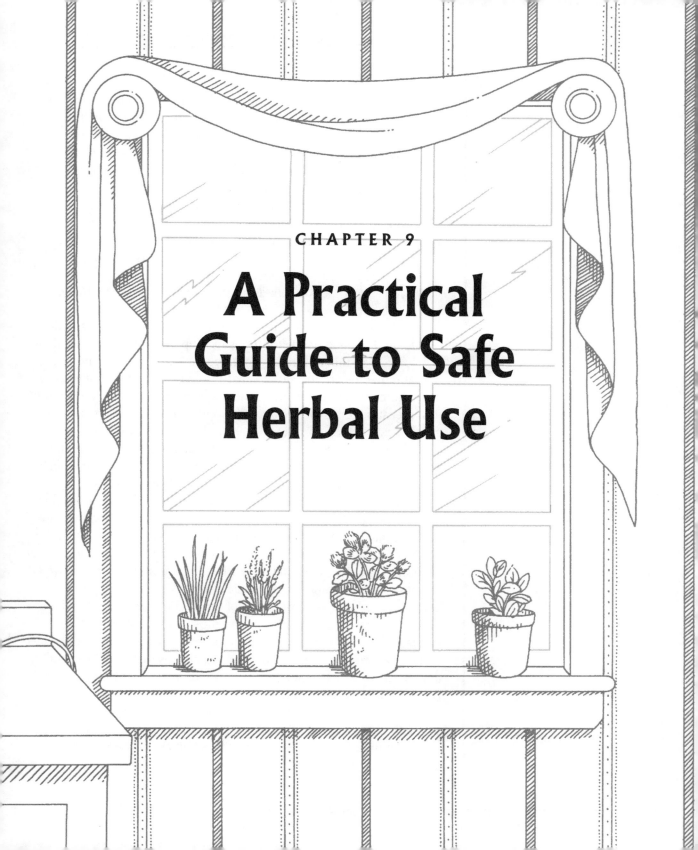

CHAPTER 9

A Practical Guide to Safe Herbal Use

Herbalism is based on relationship—relationship between plant and human, plant and planet, human and planet. Using herbs in the healing process means taking part in an ecological cycle. This offers us the opportunity to consciously be present in the living, vital world of which we are part; to invite wholeness and our world into our lives through awareness of the remedies being used. The herbs can link us into the broader context of planetary wholeness, so that whilst they are doing their physiological/medical job, we can do ours and build an awareness of the links and mutual relationships.

—DAVID HOFFMANN, *The New Holistic Herbal*

Although herbal medicines have been serving people's health and healing needs for thousands upon thousands of years, we tend to think of them as innocuous—and safe. By and large, herbal remedies are the safest way to treat most bodily dysfunctions, from the everyday minor ones, such as cuts and scrapes, colds and flus, menstrual difficulties, and childhood ailments, to more serious conditions, such as chronic arthritis and respiratory problems. Nonetheless, it must be stressed that herbs are not merely helpful plants: They can be potent medicine and, as such, are to be treated with the respect any powerful drug or agent deserves.

Today, we tend to think of herbs as "natural" forms of drugs, but they are actually *foods* that possess medicinal qualities, and they are ingested into the system (or used topically and absorbed through the skin) just as our ordinary foods are. In fact, many common foods that we don't consider to be "herbal" or healing are now being discovered to possess a wide range of beneficial properties. For example, the common blueberry—stuff of many a homemade cobbler and millions of muffins—has been found to be the most potent antioxidant (the substance that fights free radicals in the system) extant. It outdistances by far the former favorite antioxidant substances that have been highly touted. And, the substance lycopene, which is thought to reduce the risk of prostate cancer and inhibit the spread of several types of cancer, including breast cancer, lung cancer, endometrial cancer, and stomach cancer, is found in astonishing abundance in one of our most common vegetables—the ubiquitous tomato! Whoever thought

WHERE TO FIND A NATURAL HEALTH CARE PROFESSIONAL

∾ American Association of Naturopathic
    Physicians (AANP)
601 Valley Street, Suite 105
Seattle, Washington 98109
206-298-0126
Referral line: 206-298-0125
Fax: 206-298-0129

The AANP is the professional association for practitioners of naturopathic medicine.

∾ The American Herbalists Guild
Post Office Box 70
Roosevelt, Utah 84066
435-722-8434
Fax: 435-722-8452
e-mail: *ahgoffice@earthlink.net*
Web site: *http://www.healthy.net/herbalists*

The Guild represents the interests of professional
clinical herbalists of North America and is a source for
obtaining authoritative information on the therapeutic
use of herbs.

∾ American Holistic Medical Association
4101 Lake Boone Trail, Suite 201
Raleigh, North Carolina 27607
919-787-5146
Fax: 919-787-4916

∾ Herb Research Foundation (HRF)
1007 Pearl Street, Suite 200
Boulder, Colorado 80302

800-748-2617
Fax: 303-449-7849
e-mail: *rmccaleb@herbs.org*

HRF is an internationally recognized center for
herbal research and education.

∾ National Institute of Medical Herbalists (NIMH)
56 Longbrook Street
Exeter, Devon
United Kingdom EX4 6AH
011-44-39-242-6022
Fax: 011-44-39-249-8963

NIMH is a membership and certification organization for medical herbalists in the United Kingdom.

∾ National Institutes of Health (NIH)
Office of Complementary and Alternative
    Medicine (OCAM)
9000 Rockville Pike, Building 31
Bethesda, Maryland 20829
301-402-2466 or 301-402-4334

NIH and OCAM are U.S. government institutions.

∾ Ontario Herbalists Association
11 Winthrop Place
Stoney Creek, Ontario, Canada L8G 3M3
905-536-1509
Fax: 905-536-1567

spaghetti drenched in tomato sauce would be good for you? (As it turns out, the lycopene in tomatoes is released better when it is both cooked and concentrated. Those "eight great tomatoes in the itty bitty can" may one day be taken by the spoonful as an herbal remedy.) Used as foods or flavoring agents (e.g., garlic, parsley, turmeric), herbs combine with our bodies and are thus able to address both the symptoms and underlying causes of a health problem. Herbs offer the body nutrients it does not always receive—often commercially grown food is grown on depleted soil as well as doused with pesticides. Many people do not pay sufficient attention to proper nutrition because they are "too busy" or simply lack the knowledge or interest.

When considering safety, it is important to remember that herbs, when used as medicines, are essentially body balancers that help the body's entire ecosystem to heal itself.

If you are going to use herbs medicinally, there are three primary rules you should follow:

1. Do not self-diagnose. Even minor conditions could be symptoms of a serious problem. If possible, consult someone who is a natural health care specialist (see box).
2. Work closely with your health care provider. If you are under the care of a physician who is giving you prescription drugs, discuss any herbal treatments you are considering with him or her.
3. Educate yourself about herbs and their uses. Bookstore shelves are crammed with dozens of books on herbs for every purpose; some are regularly updated with new information (see box).

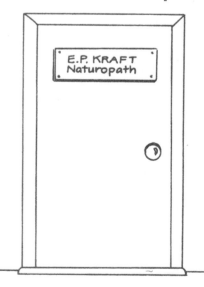

E.P. KRAFT
Naturopath

Generally speaking, herbs provide a rich variety of healing agents and—as most of them are edible plants—they are as safe as foods and have almost no side effects. Of course, one must *always* consider the individual who is taking the herbs, and for what reasons. Just as some persons are allergic to certain foods and have adverse reactions to eating, say strawberries or eggplant, one must take one's own constitutional nature into consideration.

If, for example, aspirin upsets your stomach, you would not want to take willow bark, from which aspirin is derived.

HERBAL RESOURCES

Selected Herbal Books

- *The Way of Herbs* by Michael Tierra, L.Ac., O.M.D.
- *The Healing Power of Herbs* by Michael T. Murray, N.D.
- *Earl Mindell's Herb Bible* by Earl Mindell, R.Ph., Ph.D.
- *The New Holistic Herbal* by David Hoffmann
- *The Complete Medicinal Herbal* by Penelope Ody
- *The Illustrated Encyclopedia of Natural Remedies* by C. Norman Shealy, M.D., Ph.D.
- *Natural Healing with Herbs* by Humbart Santillo, B.S., M.H.
- *Healing Plants* by Ana Nez Heatherley
- *The Woman's Book of Healing Herbs* by Sari Harrar and Sara Altshul O'Donnell
- *The Healing Herbs* by Michael Castleman

Noteworthy Herb Periodical Publications

- *Herbalgram*
  American Botanical Council
  Post Office Box 201660
  Austin, Texas
  512-926-4900

Herbalgram is the quarterly magazine of the American Botanical Council and the Herb Research Foundation.

- *American Herb Association Quarterly Newsletter*
  Contact Kathi Keville
  Post Office Box 1673
  Nevada City, California 95959

- *Medical Herbalism*
  Paul Bergner, Editor
  Post Office Box 20512
  Boulder, Colorado 80308
  303-541-9552

This bimonthly letter is primarily for herbal medical practitioners, but it is an important resource for anyone seriously interested in healing with herbs.

- *The Herb Companion*
  Interweave Press
  201 East Fourth Street
  Loveland, Colorado 80537
  800-272-2193
  Fax: 970-6678317
  e-mail: *hc@lwp.ccmail.compuserve.com*

This is a bimonthly full-color magazine "celebrating the useful plants."

The key to avoiding an adverse reaction is in moderation—both in formulation and in dosage. *Always* follow the dosage recommendations on the labels of any herbal products you buy and, if you make your own preparations be sure you have proper directions. Anything mishandled or taken to excess can cause negative side effects, but these are easy enough to avoid with proper attention and care (just as you wash your cutting board after dissecting a raw chicken to avoid contaminating your other food with bacteria). The use of common sense is as important regarding taking herbs as it is in preparing food, driving your car, working around the house, or any other area of life. Safety is never a guarantee without proper precaution.

However, as a general rule, herbs can be used freely and safely as part of one's health regimen, just as one might take a daily multiple vitamin tablet, considering it not as medicine but as a health benefit for maintenance.

Herbs in their whole form are not drugs. Therefore, do not expect them to act like drugs with which you are familiar. Modern herb-based drugs are not herbs—they are chemicals. Drugs usually treat only the *symptoms* of a problem—so you have a headache, you take a NSAID such as Tylenol or aspirin and, bingo! The headache goes away. However, the fight you just had with your spouse or your teenager or your boss, which was the real cause of your headache, is an issue not addressed by the NSAID. Herbs tend to work on the whole person, including the emotions. And some herbal remedies are specifically aimed at correcting negative emotions that result in physical dysfunction. Unlike drugs, herbal remedies are also often used in conjunction with other health-supporting methods, such as massage, aromatherapy, meditation, and the like.

Therefore, as herbal medicine works differently from prescription drugs, and as herbs themselves act as foundation nutrients for the glands and hormones, which affect the brain, they can act to support, control, and even reverse the root cause of a problem, with more long-lasting, even permanent, effect. Chronic or long-standing problems will naturally take longer treatment than new ones with which herbal treatment tends to work quickly. And as health improves with herbal support, infections and other ailments tend to decrease in proportion. It is important to remember that what did not occur overnight isn't going to be cured overnight and to allow time to work its magic of healing.

SAFETY FIRST WITH HERBS

All professional practitioners who use herbs as medicine are concerned with their safety. Jennifer Brett, N.D., chair of botanical medicine at the University of Bridgeport College of Naturopathic Medicine in Connecticut, offers these three cautionary suggestions for keeping herbal healing safe:

1. Don't use herbs with drugs that have similar active ingredients or that act on the body in similar ways. For instance, don't combine blood-thinning herbs like willow bark (from which aspirin is derived) with an anticoagulant prescription drug such as warfarin.
2. Avoid taking herbs at the same time that you take supplements or medications. Taking different types of preparations at different times of day counteracts the off chance that they might interact negatively. Ginger, for instance, can interfere with heart medications and blood thinners.
3. Avoid herbs that increase or decrease the time needed for other medications (or supplements) to be absorbed into the body. For example, licorice lengthens the time it takes prednisone to clear the body.

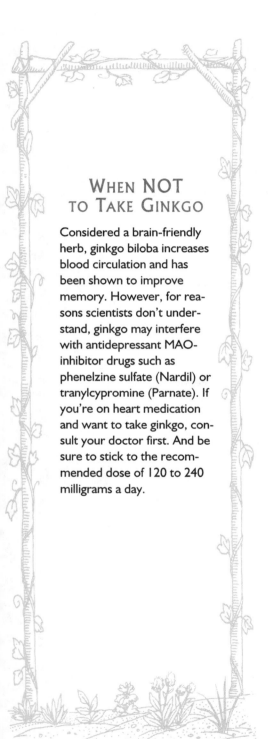

WHEN NOT TO TAKE GINKGO

Considered a brain-friendly herb, ginkgo biloba increases blood circulation and has been shown to improve memory. However, for reasons scientists don't understand, ginkgo may interfere with antidepressant MAO-inhibitor drugs such as phenelzine sulfate (Nardil) or tranylcypromine (Parnate). If you're on heart medication and want to take ginkgo, consult your doctor first. And be sure to stick to the recommended dose of 120 to 240 milligrams a day.

Specific herbs strengthen and tone specific organs and regular use may overcome any tendency to weakness in those areas. For example, hawthorn berries support the circulatory system, and a recent study has shown that horse chestnut is an excellent herb to enhance the circulation. Clinical trials in humans have shown that an extract of horse chestnut, formed into sustained-release pellets contained in capsules, effectively relieves the symptoms of chronic venous insufficiency (CVI), which is the cause of varicose veins, spider veins, and swelling in the ankles and feet. The total daily dose is 600 milligrams. The German Commission E (the world's leading authority on herb safety) states that the sustained-release form of horse chestnut extract is a safe and effective treatment for CVI. Side effects are minor and rare. Also, the extract can be used to prevent foot and ankle swelling resulting from flying long distances. Flyers who took a 600-milligram dose prior to a flight reported their swelling was significantly less than without the extract.

The German Commission E has also approved the herb butcher's broom as supportive of the circulation system, recommending a dose of 300 milligrams of the prepared product in capsule form.

Following are more examples of supportive herbs safe to take over extended periods of time:

Mullein—for the respiratory system

Meadowsweet—for the digestive system

Skullcap—for the nervous system

Nettle—for the skin

Celery seed—for the muscular and skeletal system

Raspberry leaves—for the reproductive system

Buchu—for the urinary system.

Mullein

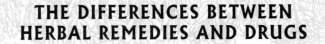

THE DIFFERENCES BETWEEN
HERBAL REMEDIES AND DRUGS

HERBAL MEDICINES	CONVENTIONAL DRUGS
Are based on entire, whole plant	Are based on isolated chemicals
Are made from natural substances	May be synthetic
Are created from the sun's energy	Are unrelated to Nature's cycle
Have few if any side effects	Always have side effects
Work slowly and subtly	Work dramatically
Enhance vitality	Deplete vitality

Herbs versus Vitamins

Although specific herbs contain specific vitamin components, herbs are *not* vitamins and should not be confused with them. The purpose of vitamins, which are extracted and concentrated, is usually to maintain health on a regular basis—to get the "minimum daily requirement," as set by the government health advisors (usually, this figure is too low). Since vitamins are concentrated substances and do not work with the body, as do herbs which are whole, they function differently. For example, if you take more vitamin C than your body can use, it will simply excrete the excess in your urine.

Herbs should not be taken like vitamins, that is, simply for maintenance of normal health. Certain herbs, that are also food—like garlic and onions—can beneficially be used on a daily basis for their health giving properties. However, therapeutic herbs work best when used only when needed and only for as long as they are needed. As the problem improves, dosage should be reduced and eventually discontinued.

Balance is the key. As herbal effects can be quite specific, you need to evaluate your need and have a clear goal in mind. When considering herbs as remedies, ask yourself the following questions:

- Is this for short- or long-term use?
- Is my problem acute (new) or chronic (long term)?
- Is this to cure a particular ailment, or is it to be a supportive treatment?
- Is this for a specific body system, such as the respiratory system, or for general body toning?
- Is this for relief of symptoms (such as a cold) or is for rebalancing (as after an illness or surgery).

SCIENTIFIC PROOF OF HERBAL SAFETY

In the 1970s, when herbal use began to rise in popularity, numerous articles appeared in medical journals and the lay press questioning the safety of herbal remedies. Since that time, herb usage has increased dramatically—but reports of toxicity have not. In a June 1992 article in the *Food and Drug Law Journal*, the results of an extensive review on herbal safety concluded that there was a lack of substantial evidence that toxic reactions to herbal products was a source of concern for public health. The study was conducted by the Herbal Research Foundation, a nonprofit organization whose membership includes experts on pharmacognosy, pharmacology, and toxicology. Their review was based on reports from the American Association of Poison Control Centers and the Centers for Disease Control in Atlanta, Georgia.

While it is true that herbs growing in the wild can cause significant toxicity, those commonly used in the United States for health purposes are considered safe (with the precautions noted in individual listings, especially concerning pregnant women who should not take any herbs). Unlike prescription drugs, which often carry long lists of contraindications and possible side effects on the inserts that come with them (if they have not been removed by the pharmacist), herbal products, being sold as "dietary supplements," require that the consumer be self-responsible, which entails self-education and awareness.

The answers to these questions will guide you in your choice of herbs as remedies. Best results are usually obtained by taking the herbal remedy (or remedies) in descending strength. For the first few days, take the full dose recommended by the manufacturer; then decrease it by half. If, for example, the label says, "one or two capsules three times a day," take two, then reduce to one. After the first week, depending on results, skip a day altogether. You can continue this on/off procedure until the condition clears and then discontinue use unless it reappears. *Never* exceed the recommended dosage. This will ensure safe use.

We can count on the safety and efficacy of herbs in ways that the newest "wonder" drug can never permit. Therapeutic herbs have *spirit* and it gives them wide-ranging properties, some of which we have only begun to recognize. Herbs are complex "personalities" that we call plants—but they have a history as old as Earth itself. They have proved themselves adaptable to environmental changes, have evolved over the millennia, and have contributed much to humankind through their interactions with us. Herbs are ancient and modern at the same time. They watched the pyramids being built—and they have watched flights to the moon. Earthlings like us, earthbound, they exemplify what is best about planet Earth.

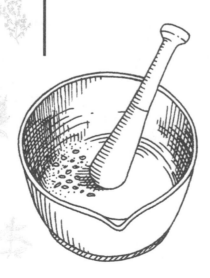

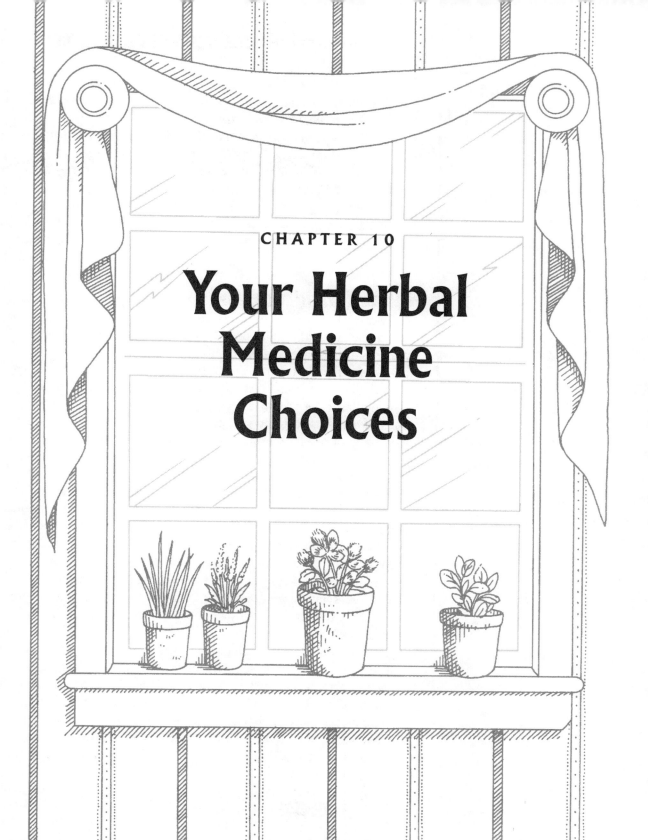

CHAPTER 10

Your Herbal Medicine Choices

The revival of interest in herbal medicine is a worldwide phenomenon. This renaissance is due in part to the public's growing concern over the side effects of pharmaceutical drugs, as well as the impersonal and often demeaning experience of modern health care practices. But above all this is the fact that herbal medicine is presently achieving renewed recognition as having unique medicinal value as a natural healer.

—Mark Blumenthal, Executive Director of the American Botanical Council

What Constitutes an Herb?

The word *herb*, as used in herbal remedies, is also known as "botanical medicine" and, in Europe, "phytotherapy" or "phytomedicine." All of these terms simply mean that a plant or plant part is used to make a medicinal preparation. An herb can be the entire plant or any or some of its parts: leaf, flower, stem, seed, root, fruit, bark.

One particular way to categorize herbs is by looking at what kinds of ailments respond to their use. Another way is to look at how many of our modern-day drugs are based on herbal components. These synthesized substances, now known as drugs, have been separated out from the whole plant by various means.

One of the first modern drugs to be isolated from a plant was morphine, which was first identified in 1803 by the German Friedrich Seturner. Using opium poppy plants, he extracted white crystals from them using techniques that soon became routine. As a result, aconitine was made from monkshood, emetine from ipecacuanha, atropine from deadly nightshade, and quinine from Peruvian bark. All of these synthesized compounds, categorized as alkaloids, were extremely potent and previously could be obtained only from the raw plants themselves.

The original breakthrough of converting the actual plant into a "pill" came in 1852, when salicin, which had been identified as one of the active ingredients in willow bark, was artificially synthesized for the first time. Later, acetylsalicylic acid, what we now know as aspirin, was chemically modified because the product proved to upset the stomach lining of in some people. In 1899, acetylsalicylic acid was launched into the marketplace as aspirin by the Bayer drug company.

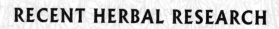

RECENT HERBAL RESEARCH

INSTITUTION	STUDY FOR	REMEDY
Harvard Medical School	Antioxidant	Ginkgo
New York Presbyterian Hospital	Pain relief	Aromatherapy
University of Texas Center for Alternative Medicine Research in Cancer, Houston	Cancer Prevention	Green tea, shark cartilage, ginseng, mistletoe
University of California, San Francisco, Osher Center	Treating chemotherapy side effects	Chinese herbal medicine

Since then, a hundred years ago, plant extracts have become commonplace on pharmacy shelves. Ephedrine preparations from *ma huang* are available both in over-the-counter and prescription forms.

For centuries, the plant Indian snakeroot was used in Ayurvedic medicine for a range of problems, including anxiety, headache, fevers, and snakebites. Mahatma Gandhi was reputed to drink a cup of snakeroot tea at bedtime if he had had a busy day and felt over-stimulated. Western herbalists valued it as a powerful tranquilizer and also used it to treat high blood pressure.

Then, in 1947, scientists extracted the alkaloid reserpine from snakeroot and began marketing a drug called Serpasil for high blood pressure. This drug proved to have many unpleasant side effects, and in the 1950s, a new tranquilizer was developed from the herb. This has always been a prescription-only drug in the United States, but in other parts of the world, including Europe and Asia, snakeroot in its natural state continues to be widely used as a soothing tea and tranquilizer.

To date, out of the approximately five hundred thousand plant species on Earth, only about five thousand have been thoroughly studied for their medicinal value. This means that there is still a vast number of plants that may hold hidden within their leaves, seeds, flowers, fruits, and roots the cures for some of humanity's most perplexing diseases, such as cancer, AIDS, diabetes, or other illnesses today considered incurable. This fact alone should make us treat all plant life, and especially herbal plant life, with great respect.

The Value of Plants in Health and Healing

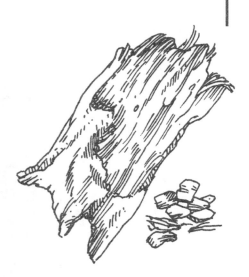

In many parts of the world, herbs are the only option available to treat medical problems. Because herbs take an indirect route to the bloodstream, their effects are usually slower and more subtle than purified drugs administered by a doctor writing a prescription. In Colonial America, and even into the 19th century, housewives had extensive herbal knowledge of home remedies. However, much herbal knowledge has been lost because it was not passed down from generation to generation, as it was in traditional cultures. As the 20th century medical advances became more and more dramatic, the populace assumed a "doctor knows best" attitude, giving up responsibility for and control of their health care. Fortunately, this is now changing. Today, Americans are rediscovering herbal healing with unprecedented enthusiasm. Recent studies show that more than 75 percent of Americans now use some form of alternative healing for their health care, with the result that herbal remedies have become immensely popular as natural health promoters, and as complements to over-the-counter drugstore medicines and prescription drugs as well. Even the American academic establishment is getting into the herbal medicine act, with major U.S. research centers now investigating the healing potential of herbs and other alternative medical approaches.

An established theory is that herbs can ward off cancer by their indirect stimulation of the immune system, but in recent years researchers have begun identifying plant components that are actively anticancer. Herbs contain scores of these biologically active chemicals, which may one day be proved to have therapeutic use. Several anticancer drugs have already been derived from plants, the most notable of which is Taxol, from the Pacific yew tree.

Another is milk thistle, which has been studied at Case Western Reserve University in Cleveland. The studies indicate that most of these plant chemicals block carcinogens from damaging healthy cells and triggering the growth of the tumor. They may also inhibit the reproduction of tumor cells. Already, studies of garlic and onions indicate that they contain chemicals that cause the carcinogens to be excreted from the body before they can cause harmful effects.

The metabolism of nature's intelligence takes place on the level of the neuroreceptors in the human body, which serve as a link between the physical body and the environment in which it lives. The human body possesses a multitude of neuroreceptors that are responsive to biological substances found in herbs. These substances have the capacity of targeting specific receptors within the body. Thus, the health and balance of the body—the yin/yang in Chinese terms—is restored through the plant's influence.

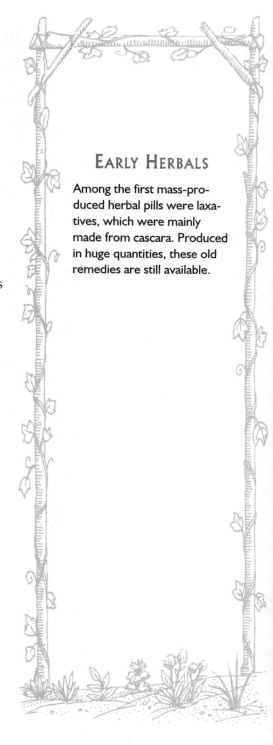

EARLY HERBALS

Among the first mass-produced herbal pills were laxatives, which were mainly made from cascara. Produced in huge quantities, these old remedies are still available.

Whole Plant Extracts versus Standardized Extracts versus Drugs

As American health care consumers increase their purchase of herbal products as natural alternatives to drugs, the standardizing of separate herbal constituents for guaranteed potency is becoming common. Today's herbal product manufacturers are doing this more and more as they enter the drug-oriented health care market.

Standardization is a divisive issue among herbalists. The purists want to see only the fresh, whole herb used. The producers, who of necessity must be realists, are forced to deal with government rules and regulations of their products. It's a case of fitting a square peg into a round hole, as government regulators and the orthodox medical establishment attempt to fit herbal remedies into the existing laboratory drug mold. There is no doubt that American consumers need and will demand safety standards. In addition, few of them—only the most dedicated—will go out into the wild and gather their own herbal plants (of course, after learning to correctly identify them) and then process them into pills, powders, poultices, ointments, oils, and other homemade forms.

These factors combine to make standardization popular, even if controversial. According to Linda Rector Page, N.D., Ph.D., standardization is a mistake. In her book, *Herbal Healing*, she says:

> As a naturopath and traditional herbalist, I believe that standardization short-changes the full spectrum of whole-herb healing. Throughout the ages and from many cultures and traditions, herbalists have effectively used whole herbs for whole bodies with immense success that rivals modern day allopathic medicine. . . . Yet, in the modern health care world, laboratory yardsticks are the only measurements science understands or government approves. . . . Standardizing a so-called "active ingredient" in a drug-like approach neglects one of the main features of whole herbs. . . . their internal complexity. Single herbs contain dozens of natural chemical constituents working synergistically. . . . the natural herb [is] in correct and balanced ratios with all its constituents.

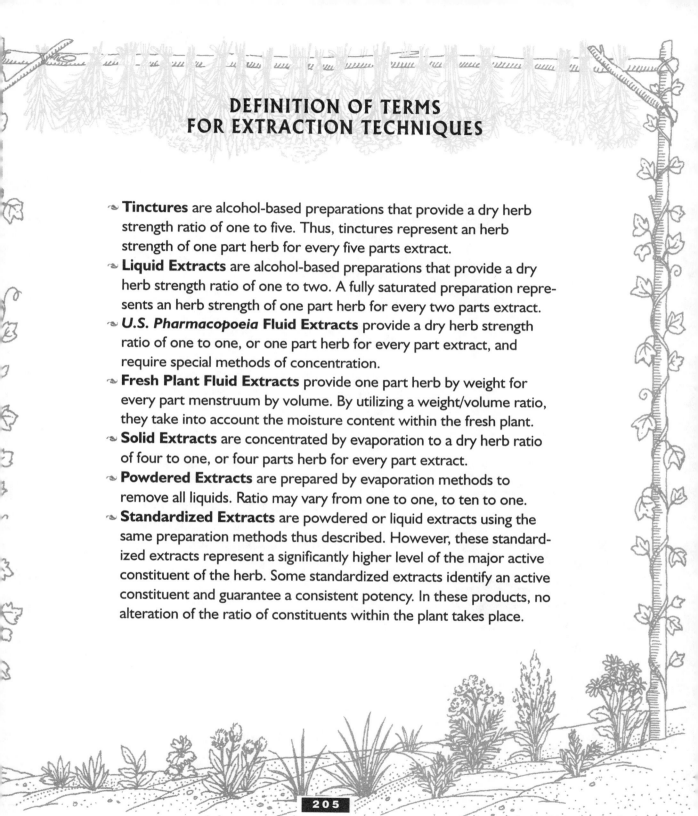

DEFINITION OF TERMS
FOR EXTRACTION TECHNIQUES

- **Tinctures** are alcohol-based preparations that provide a dry herb strength ratio of one to five. Thus, tinctures represent an herb strength of one part herb for every five parts extract.
- **Liquid Extracts** are alcohol-based preparations that provide a dry herb strength ratio of one to two. A fully saturated preparation represents an herb strength of one part herb for every two parts extract.
- **U.S. Pharmacopoeia Fluid Extracts** provide a dry herb strength ratio of one to one, or one part herb for every part extract, and require special methods of concentration.
- **Fresh Plant Fluid Extracts** provide one part herb by weight for every part menstruum by volume. By utilizing a weight/volume ratio, they take into account the moisture content within the fresh plant.
- **Solid Extracts** are concentrated by evaporation to a dry herb ratio of four to one, or four parts herb for every part extract.
- **Powdered Extracts** are prepared by evaporation methods to remove all liquids. Ratio may vary from one to one, to ten to one.
- **Standardized Extracts** are powdered or liquid extracts using the same preparation methods thus described. However, these standardized extracts represent a significantly higher level of the major active constituent of the herb. Some standardized extracts identify an active constituent and guarantee a consistent potency. In these products, no alteration of the ratio of constituents within the plant takes place.

Thus, common drugs and standardized herbal remedies utilizing only limited constituents of a plant do not have the holistic properties that the whole plant extracts do, and therefore they do not act the same. Some standardized herbal preparations favor a particular active constituent of a plant over other components. Common drugs synthesize a chemical similar to an active plant constituent. Both can have potent effects, but only at the expense of the whole.

By contrast, whole plant extracts—properly and scientifically prepared under meticulous conditions—provide the complete range of the plant's inner chemistry, which, being synergistic, acts with the body in a holistic way.

Standardization is seen by some herbal product companies, especially those whose main focus has been vitamins, as an effective means to challenge the mainstream drug company monopoly, by accurately measuring and guaranteeing potency of one or more active constituents of a plant for medical use.

It is also a way of dealing with FDA regulations regarding measurability and guidelines for listing active ingredients on labels. FDA regulations were never intended to deal with the complexities or broad-based effects of herbal remedies, so changes must eventually be made to accommodate them. This task will not be an easy one, but it is one that must be accomplished.

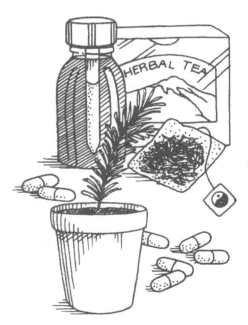

How to Obtain Healing Herbs

There are three ways to obtain healing herbs: gather them in the wild, grow them yourself, or buy them. Since most people will choose to buy ready-made preparations in their health food stores or from mail-order sources rather than either gathering or growing them, here are some pointers to use when buying medicinal herbs:

- Whenever possible, buy herbs that are organically grown or wildcrafted (grown in their natural habitat). Buy locally grown fresh-dried herbs.
- If buying bulk herbs, test a sample by rubbing some between your fingers to check the smell. Even dried herbs when crushed give off strong evidence of their volatile oils, and so potency is easily evident.

THE FIRST HERBAL PRODUCTS COMPANY

Most people think of the Shakers as designers and builders of excellently crafted furniture that is beautiful as well as practical, but few know that they were the first people to sell herbal remedies in packages. They invented the pill as a form of medicine, it being more convenient than the old-fashioned powders. The Shakers were the first in this country to produce herbs for hospitals and for the pharmaceutical market. Their products were known in the commercial world for their quality. France's Professor C. S. Rafinesque said in 1851 that the Shakers had, "the best medicinal gardens in the United States. [They] cultivate and collect a great variety of medical plants. They sell them cheap, fresh, and genuine."

The Shakers developed a thriving business in medicinal herbs. At first, they used herbs themselves in their communities, but they felt a commitment to provide their knowledge to others, and so they began to sell little packets of their prepared herbs, which became extremely popular. In their 1831 shipping record, there is an order of medicinal herbs to Charles Whitlaw, botanist of London, totaling $895.65.

Their devotion to detail led them to speak of a "consecrated industry." This implies that there was a spiritual component to their herbal business, which became the basis of their very substantial prosperity.

The first Shaker herb catalog was printed in Albany in 1831 and listed 120 varieties of wild herbs with medicinal uses. Adding roots, barks, berries, and seeds of many plants, the number of items totaled 142. In addition, there were twelve medicinal preparations, along with a listing of the disorders they were intended to cure.

For their plant names, the Shakers used the various *Manuals of Botany, 1817–1840* by Amos Eaton. Prior to the publication of Torey and Gray's *Flora of North America* (1838–1843), Professor Eaton was the leading authority on the botany of the northeastern states. One of the biggest moneymakers and a chief product of the Shakers was dandelion (used in Dr. Corbett's Shaker Sarsaparilla Syrup).

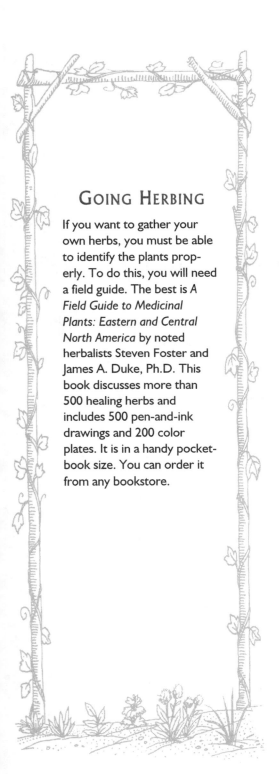

GOING HERBING

If you want to gather your own herbs, you must be able to identify the plants properly. To do this, you will need a field guide. The best is *A Field Guide to Medicinal Plants: Eastern and Central North America* by noted herbalists Steven Foster and James A. Duke, Ph.D. This book discusses more than 500 healing herbs and includes 500 pen-and-ink drawings and 200 color plates. It is in a handy pocketbook size. You can order it from any bookstore.

- Never stint on quality. Buy the best available. Bargain herbs are usually adulterated. More costly products from reputable companies are a better choice because the growing/gathering/preparation/storage phases of the process are supported by experience and quality control.
- When choosing packaged herbs, buy from a company that specializes in herbs, not one that is primarily a supplier of vitamins or other supplements. Herbal companies tend to be devotees of their product and have a high level of integrity in handling and preparation.
- Make sure any product you buy is tightly sealed and has been kept away from excess light and heat. Check the expiration date.
- Ask your herbal consultant or health care practitioner what brands he or she recommends (see Chapter 9 for information on how to find a herbal practitioner).
- Do not rely on information about herbs from a clerk in a health food store or pharmacy, especially if it is part of a large chain store. Ask to see the buyer of herbal products or the store manager if you want information. You can also ask whether they have a qualified herbalist on staff or can recommend someone who practices herbalism locally. Such a person would likely be a regular customer.

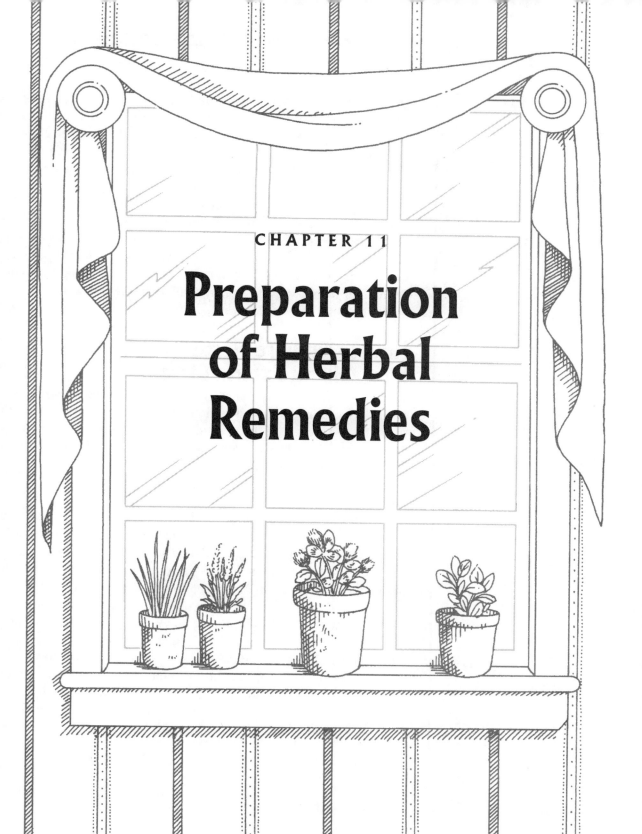

CHAPTER 11

Preparation
of Herbal
Remedies

S tress is a part of life that is, unfortunately, often unavoidable. You may not be able to avoid stress, but there are some things you can do to help yourself cope better when life presents a challenge. Diet, exercise, and sleep are, of course, very important components of a healthy lifestyle. Herbal remedies can be another ally in this war against stress.

Herbs can improve digestion, aid relaxation, and improve mood. They can also be used as a delicious addition to food or drink. The preparations and recipes in this chapter are designed to help you through some of the roadblocks ahead. With proper use, experimentation will help you find the remedy that is right for you. Remember to seek advice from a qualified professional if a problem persists.

How to Prepare Herbs for Internal and External Use

There are many ways to prepare herbs for use. Different herbs call for different techniques. To determine the best herbal preparation for your situation, you must first consider the desired result. The following section provides descriptions and examples of the most common types of preparations.

Bolus

A bolus is a suppository or internal poultice used in the rectum or vagina. It draws out toxins and is the carrier of healing agents. A bolus is made by adding powdered herbs to cocoa butter, creating a thick, firm consistency. The mixture is usually placed in the refrigerator to harden and is then brought to room temperature before use. A bolus can be inserted into the rectum to treat hemorrhoids and cysts, or into the vagina to treat infections, irritations, and tumors. It is usually applied at night when the cocoa butter will melt with body heat, thus releasing the herbs. The most frequently used herbs in a bolus are astringent herbs (such as white oak bark or bayberry bark), demulcent healing herbs (such as comfrey or slippery elm), or antibiotic herbs (such as garlic, chaparral, or goldenseal).

Capsules

Herbs are also available in gelatin-coated capsules. To ensure the herbs will be safe and pure and prepared by chemists trained in herbal science, be sure that you purchase capsules from a reliable company. Take capsules with 8 ounces of pure water or herbal tea.

Compress

A compress is used when herbs too strong to be taken internally need to be used for healing. Compresses are for external use and can be extremely effective because the active parts of the herb reach the affected area without being altered by the digestive process. The effects of an herbal compress are similar to those of an ointment, with the added advantage of therapeutic heat. A compress is usually made from an infusion or decoction, which is used to soak a linen or muslin cloth. The cloth is then placed on the affected area, where it can be held in place by a bandage or plastic wrap. Compresses can be hot or cold and are generally milder than poultices. The compress allows the herbs to be slowly absorbed in small amounts by the body. It is generally used in cases of injury, contusions, swellings, pains, colds, and flu. It helps to stimulate the circulatory and lymphatic systems.

To prepare a compress, add 1 or 2 heaping tablespoons of the herb(s) to 1 cup of water and bring to a boil. Dip a sterile cotton pad, gauze, or cloth into the strained liquid, drain off any excess, then place the warm compress on the affected area. It is usually beneficial to cover the compress with a piece of woolen material to hold in the heat. If using on a small child, the compress should be bandaged into place. After the compress has cooled, replace it with another hot one.

A basic example is a ginger compress. To make a ginger compress, grate 2 ounces of fresh ginger root and squeeze its juice into a pint of hot water until the water turns yellow. Apply the compress, having constant hot replacement towels ready as soon as the original cools. A ginger compress is used to stimulate the circulation of blood and lymph, to relieve colic, to reduce internal inflammation, and to restore warmth to cold joints.

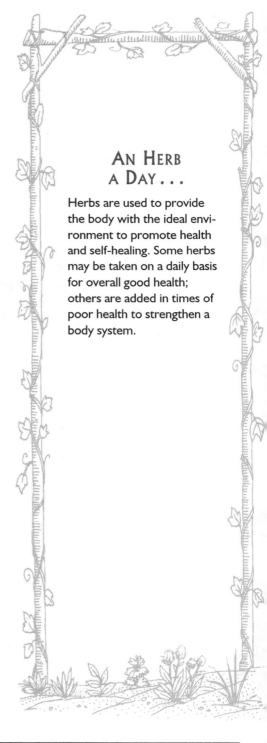

AN HERB A DAY...

Herbs are used to provide the body with the ideal environment to promote health and self-healing. Some herbs may be taken on a daily basis for overall good health; others are added in times of poor health to strengthen a body system.

Decoction

To decoct means "to extract to flavor or essence of something by boiling." The word *decoction* is used to describe the extract obtained by the boiling process. Decoctions are valuable because they contain an herb's essential mineral salts and alkaloids. The roots, twigs, berries, seeds, and bark of a plant are boiled in water. The liquid is then strained and taken with honey or brown sugar as prescribed. Decoctions are used when the root or bark is not soluble in water but will release its ingredients after simmering for five to 20 minutes.

To prepare a decoction, place a teaspoon of the dried herb in an enamel or glass container with 1 cup of pure water. Boil the mixture—for five minutes if the material is finely shredded; 20 minutes if the herb is hard or woody. It is sometimes helpful if the plant is first soaked in cold water and then boiled. Always strain the decoction while it's hot.

Essential Oils

Essential oils are often used in other therapies, such as aromatherapy. A plant's essential oils are those that contain its essence or some of its most active principles. Essential oils are useful for making tinctures and ointments.

Extracts

An extract is a concentrated form of an herb that is obtained by mixing the herb with an appropriate solvent (such as alcohol and/or water). Herbal extracts are usually made from stimulating herbs, such as cayenne, and antispasmodic herbs, such as lobelia. Extracts are used topically to treat strained muscles and ligaments or for the relief of arthritis and other inflammations.

Extracts can be made by putting four ounces of dried herbs or 8 ounces of fresh, bruised herbs into a jar or bottle with a tight-fitting lid. Add 1 pint of vinegar, alcohol, or massage oil. Over time, the liquid will extract the medicinal properties of the herbs.

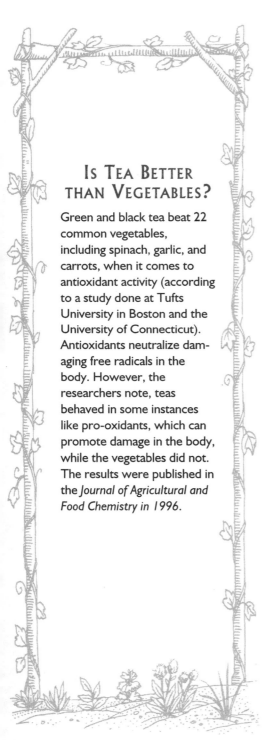

IS TEA BETTER THAN VEGETABLES?

Green and black tea beat 22 common vegetables, including spinach, garlic, and carrots, when it comes to antioxidant activity (according to a study done at Tufts University in Boston and the University of Connecticut). Antioxidants neutralize damaging free radicals in the body. However, the researchers note, teas behaved in some instances like pro-oxidants, which can promote damage in the body, while the vegetables did not. The results were published in the *Journal of Agricultural and Food Chemistry* in 1996.

It will take approximately four days to get a potent extract if the herbs are powdered, and about 15 days if the herbs are whole or cut. You must shake the bottle once or twice daily. If olive or almond oils are used in the extract, a little vitamin E can be added as a preservative. Making an extract with oil is useful if it is to be used for massage purposes. Using alcohol extract (vodka or gin), or rubbing alcohol (for external use only), allows the liquid to evaporate quickly, leaving the herbs on the skin while providing a cooling sensation.

Hydrotherapy: The Herb Bath

The use of water for treatment of illness, otherwise known as hydrotherapy, is extremely popular in Europe, where health spas are commonplace. The good news is that you don't have to go to a spa to enjoy the benefits of hydrotherapy! You can indulge in an herbal bath in your own home. To make a decoction for a full bath, anywhere from several ounces to a pound of plant parts should be sewn into a linen bag and boiled in a quart or more of water. The water is then added to the bath. You can also put the bag into the bath to extract more of its properties, or you can use it as a washcloth. Bathing with herbs accelerates their absorption through the skin. It makes them especially effective for circulation troubles, swelling from broken bones, arthritis, and gout. The therapeutic effects of herbs result from inhaling the steam and from the herbs entering the bloodstream through the skin. For example, an oatmeal bath works topically on eczema, and a chamomile bath soothes the skin and relaxes the body. The calming effects alone make herbal baths a wonderful prescription for relaxation.

Infusion

An infusion is an extract made from herbs with medicinal components in their flowers, leaves, and stems. It is made by pouring hot liquid over a crude or powdered herb and then allowing the mixture to steep. This extracts the herb's active ingredients and also minimizes the loss of volatile elements. Infusions are prepared much like teas, but they are steeped longer and are considerably stronger.

About Tea

In her book, *The Herbal Tea Garden*, Marietta Marshall Marcin provides the following definition of tea:

> In the narrowest sense of the word, tea refers to the leaves or flower buds of shrubs in the genus that was named *Thea sinensis* by Swedish botanist, Carolus Linnaeus. Since *Thea sinensis* tea is a close relative of the camellis flower, it is sometimes referred to as *Camellia thea* or *Camellia sinensis*. Broadly speaking, however, tea is any drink made from steeping fragrant leaves, berries, seeds, flowers, roots, or bark in boiling water.

She explains that many different *Thea sinensis* teas, such as black, green, orange, pekoe, and oolong are made from leaves of the same plant. However, they differ in the degree of fermentation they have undergone during processing.

The normal ratio used in preparing an infusion is about ½ to 1 ounce of an herb to 1 pint of water. Use a glass, enamel, or porcelain pot, and steep the herbs for about 10 to 20 minutes, covered with a tight-fitting lid to prevent evaporation. For general use, strain the infusion and drink it lukewarm or cool, but to induce sweating and break up a cold of cough, drink it hot. Remember that infusions have a short shelf life, so don't let them spoil.

Inhalations

Warm moist air can relieve many respiratory problems and allow the healing properties of herbs to enter the bloodstream through the lungs. To prepare an inhalation, fill a large bowl half full of steaming water, and add an herbal infusion or decoction, or two to three drops of an essential oil.

Oils

Oil extracts are a useful way of preparing a concentrate. Herbal oils are very useful when ointments or compresses are not practical. Oils are prepared first by macerating and pounding fresh or dried herbs. Olive or sesame oil is then added, 2 ounces of herb to 1 pint of oil. The mixture should then be allowed to sit in a warm place for about four days before it is used. A shortcut is to gently heat the herbs and oil in a pan for one hour. The oil can then be strained and bottled. Adding a small amount of vitamin E will preserve the oil. Oil extracts are usually made from aromatic herbs such as eucalyptus, peppermint, spearmint, and spices.

Ointments

Ointments are used on the skin when the active ingredients of an herb are needed for extended periods of time, such as in the event of injury, contusion, and effusion. Ointments stay on the skin and accelerate the healing process. To prepare an ointment at home, bring 1 or 2 heaping tablespoons of the herb(s) and a good helping of petroleum jelly to a boil (there are petroleum jelly products made from natural sources that can be used). Then stir and strain the mixture. After it has cooled, store it in a jar for use when needed.

Poultices

An herbal poultice is a soft, moist, hot mass of fresh, ground, or powdered herbs applied to the body medicinally. A poultice is put directly on the skin to relieve inflammation, blood poisoning, venomous bites, eruptions, boils, abscesses, and to promote proper cleansing and healing of the affected area. Many herbs contain ingredients necessary to draw out infections, toxins, and foreign bodies embedded in the skin. Plantain and marshmallow are great pain relievers, and they also stop muscle spasms. Cayenne is mixed with herbs such as lobelia, valerian, catnip, and echinacea to promote stimulation and cleansing.

To prepare a poultice, moisten herbs with hot water, apple cider vinegar, herbal tea, a liniment, or a tincture. Whatever liquid you use, make sure that it is hot. Cleanse the affected area with an antiseptic and then oil the skin before applying the hot poultice.

Powders

Powders are simply fresh herbal agents that have been crushed into fine particles. Herbs in powder form can be taken in a capsule, in water, in herbal teas, or sprinkled on food. Using powdered herbs is a good way to slowly introduce herbs into your system. This allows your body time to adjust. For external use, powdered herbs can be mixed with oil, petroleum jelly, a little water, or aloe vera juice and applied to the skin to treat wounds, inflammation, and contusions.

Salves

Salves are similar to ointments. A salve is made by covering fresh or dried herbs with water, bringing the mixture to a boil, and letting it simmer for 30 minutes. The water is strained off and added to an equal amount of olive oil or safflower oil. Simmer the oil/water mixture until the water has evaporated and nothing but the oil remains. Add enough beeswax to achieve the desired consistency and pour it into a dark glass jar with a tight lid. If stored well, salves will last up to a year.

HOW LONG TO USE HERBS

One of the important factors in purchasing herbs is to determine whether you'll be using the compound therapeutically or as a tonic. Therapeutic herbs are best to take for short periods of time—one to four weeks. Tonic herbs, on the other hand, are used to alter deep imbalances within the body and are used for much longer periods, up to six months.

It is also important to apply the principle of "rest/activity" when using herbs. In general, they recommend that you use herbs six days with one day off; six months with one month off. Each period of rest from herbal usage allows the effects of the herbs to become integrated into the body's physiology.

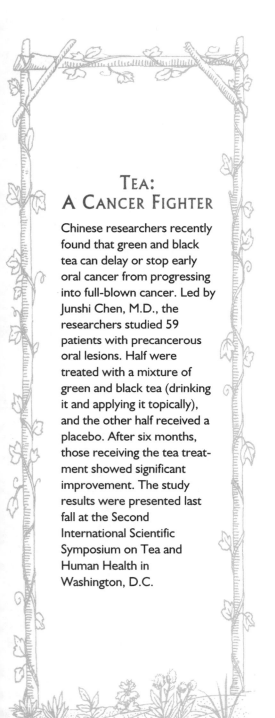

TEA: A CANCER FIGHTER

Chinese researchers recently found that green and black tea can delay or stop early oral cancer from progressing into full-blown cancer. Led by Junshi Chen, M.D., the researchers studied 59 patients with precancerous oral lesions. Half were treated with a mixture of green and black tea (drinking it and applying it topically), and the other half received a placebo. After six months, those receiving the tea treatment showed significant improvement. The study results were presented last fall at the Second International Scientific Symposium on Tea and Human Health in Washington, D.C.

Syrups

An herbal syrup is ideal for treating coughs, mucus congestion, bronchial catarrh, and sore throats because of its coating ability, which keeps the herbs in direct contact with the affected area. Syrups are especially good for children and people with sensitive palates. To make a syrup, add about 2 ounces of herbs to 1 quart of water and gently boil it down to 1 pint. While still warm, add 2 ounces of honey and/or glycerine. Licorice and wild cherry bark are commonly used in syrups as flavors and therapeutic agents. Other common choices are comfrey, anise seed, fennel, and Irish moss. Try an herbal syrup instead of a drugstore brand and decide for yourself which is more effective, and just plain healthier.

Tinctures

Tinctures are solutions of concentrated herbal extracts made with alcohol instead of water. They are more highly concentrated than infusions and decoctions and have a longer shelf life. Tinctures are usually made with strong herbs that are not taken as teas. They are also useful for distasteful herbs and those that need to be taken over an extended period of time. Tinctures are convenient for external application.

A tincture can be made by combining 4 ounces of powdered or cut herbs with 1 pint of alcohol, such as vodka or brandy. Those who do not drink alcohol can make tinctures using warm (but not boiled) vinegar; use wine or apple vinegar, but not the white variety. Allow the tincture to steep for two to four weeks, shaking every few days to encourage alcohol absorption of the herb's medicinal properties. In four weeks, strain the herbs out of the liquid. Store in a cool place out of the reach of children.

ON TINCTURES

In a generic sense, the word *tincture* refers to a liquid extract made from an herb that has been dissolved in a solvent such as grain alcohol, glycerin, water, or, rarely, another liquid. More specifically, *tincture* can be used to refer to alcoholic extracts only; glycerin-based extracts can be referred to as glycerites.

These concentrated forms of an herb's active chemicals offer several advantages over other herbal preparations. The bottles are easy to carry and need no refrigeration. The concentrated form makes it easier to take large doses. They keep for years and are easy for the body to assimilate—in fact, tinctures are often absorbed up to 40 percent better because the herb's active components have been separated from the plant's indigestible cellulose and starch.

Most tinctures on the market are alcohol based because alcohol best extracts most compounds and carries them most efficiently into the body. But don't worry: Four average doses a day usually contain less than 1 teaspoon of alcohol. And the amount of alcohol contained in an adult dose is less than that found in a ripe banana, according to Mindy Green, director of educational services for the Herb Research Foundation in Boulder, Colorado.

Teas

Herbal teas, also called infusions or tisanes, are a simple and delicious way of extracting the flavor and healing properties from herbs. They can be made with fresh or dried herbs and may be sweetened with a little honey, licorice, or slices of fresh ginger. Teas will stay fresh in the refrigerator for up to 24 hours.

Herbal teas are a very popular way to use herbs. The teas can be for relaxation, medicinal purposes, or simply for enjoyment. There are many different kinds of herbal teas, but the basic recipe is generally the same. Usually, you use 1 teaspoon dried or 2 teaspoons fresh herb to each cup of water. Put the herb into a pot or cup. Add boiling water, cover with a lid, and let steep for 10 to 15 minutes. Strain and drink as required.

Possibly the most common reason for drinking herbal tea is for relaxation. The body's nervous system can sometimes become overloaded. This is due to the "fight or flight" mechanism of the sympathetic nervous system. In reaction to a stressor, the body's basic response is one of a physical nature. The heart and lungs become more active, and processes such as digestion and elimination are suppressed. If the body is in this state for a prolonged period of time, the body's natural rhythm is thrown off balance. This leads to a state of stress. If this state is not attended to, other systems of the body may begin to suffer, not to mention one's emotions. Herbal teas can help us deal with this stress. There are many herbs that have relaxing and soothing qualities. The following section offers many recipes to choose from, including teas for medicinal purposes.

HERBAL TEA CAUTION

- Avoid all strong herbal teas during the first three months of pregnancy.
- Do not give peppermint or sage tea to children under four years of age.
- Avoid ready-made herbal mixes that contain sugar.

COCKLEBUR TEA (FOR DIARRHEA)

4 cocklebur pods

Wash the burs and put them and 2 cups cold water in a pan; cover with a lid. Place on heat and boil for 4 or 5 minutes. Strain and add enough water to make 2 cups of liquid. Take by sips for diarrhea.

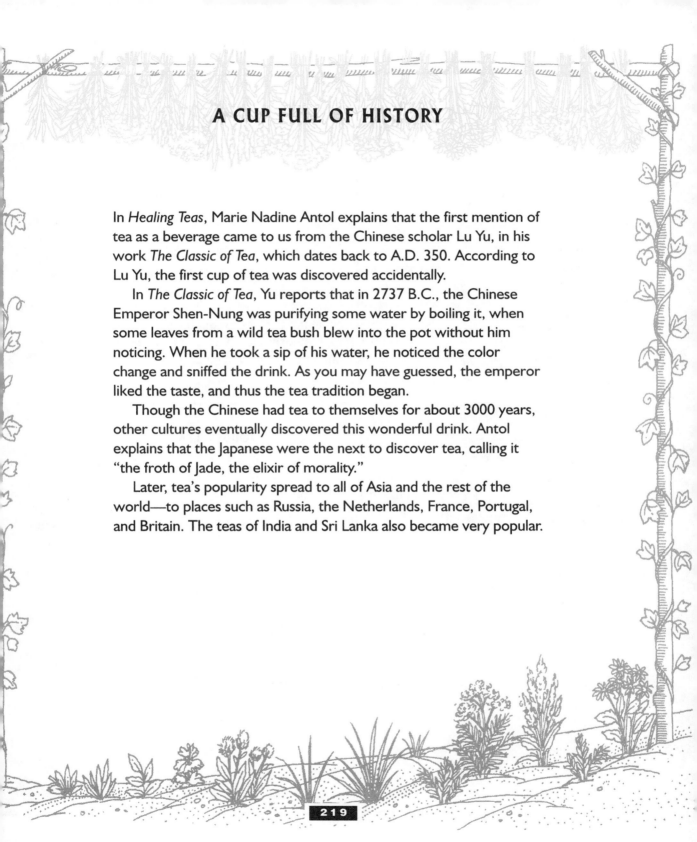

A CUP FULL OF HISTORY

In *Healing Teas*, Marie Nadine Antol explains that the first mention of tea as a beverage came to us from the Chinese scholar Lu Yu, in his work *The Classic of Tea*, which dates back to A.D. 350. According to Lu Yu, the first cup of tea was discovered accidentally.

In *The Classic of Tea*, Yu reports that in 2737 B.C., the Chinese Emperor Shen-Nung was purifying some water by boiling it, when some leaves from a wild tea bush blew into the pot without him noticing. When he took a sip of his water, he noticed the color change and sniffed the drink. As you may have guessed, the emperor liked the taste, and thus the tea tradition began.

Though the Chinese had tea to themselves for about 3000 years, other cultures eventually discovered this wonderful drink. Antol explains that the Japanese were the next to discover tea, calling it "the froth of Jade, the elixir of morality."

Later, tea's popularity spread to all of Asia and the rest of the world—to places such as Russia, the Netherlands, France, Portugal, and Britain. The teas of India and Sri Lanka also became very popular.

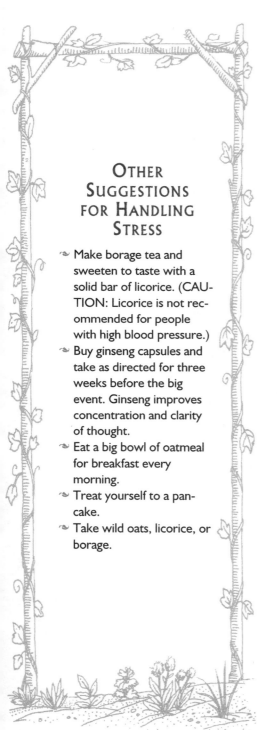

OTHER SUGGESTIONS FOR HANDLING STRESS

- Make borage tea and sweeten to taste with a solid bar of licorice. (CAUTION: Licorice is not recommended for people with high blood pressure.)
- Buy ginseng capsules and take as directed for three weeks before the big event. Ginseng improves concentration and clarity of thought.
- Eat a big bowl of oatmeal for breakfast every morning.
- Treat yourself to a pancake.
- Take wild oats, licorice, or borage.

DESERT WILLOW TEA

2 teaspoons dried desert willow leaves
1 teaspoon dried, finely chopped echinacea root

Bring 1 cup water to near boiling. Put the leaves into a bowl or pan and pour the water over them. Cover tightly and let stand for 30 minutes. Strain and keep the liquid covered in the refrigerator—do not use it after 48 hours. Make up a new batch as needed.

This tea is good for yeast infections and other problems brought on by taking antibiotics. Sip throughout the day, taking no more than 4 tablespoons in 24 hours. The tea can also be used as a douche for vaginal itching.

DODDER TEA

1 teaspoon dried dodder

Use a rounded teaspoon of dried dodder in a cup of hot water. This makes a good laxative. It can also be used for lymph node swellings, inflammation of the spleen, or liver problems; if so, it should be taken in small amounts ($^1/_2$ teaspoon) several times a day.

INDIGO TEA (TO STOP VOMITING)

Make a basic tea from indigo roots. Let it cool and add a few cubes of ice. Take sips to stop vomiting.

LEMON AND MINT TEA

¹/₂ teaspoon chopped lemongrass
¹/₂ teaspoon crushed mint (your favorite kind)

Put the herbs in a tea ball or spoon and place in a cup. Fill the cup with hot water, cover, and steep for 10 minutes. Take for headache, relaxation, or just to enjoy. This can also be made as iced tea.

ROSEMARY TEA

Make a basic tea from rosemary to relieve a tension headache.

CHAMOMILE TEA

1 teaspoon dried or 2 teaspoons fresh flowerheads
1 cup boiling water

This tea promotes relaxation and can be used to soothe restless babies and children. Inhaling the steam from this tea reduces the effects of nasal irritants and soothes symptoms of hay fever. You can also use it in the bath for relaxation.

LEMON BALM TEA

1 teaspoon fresh leaves and flowers
1 cup of boiling water

This tea aids relaxation and digestion; it is often used for irritable bowels, nervous indigestion, anxiety, and depression. It also encourages a clear mind. Drink 1 cup up to four times a day.

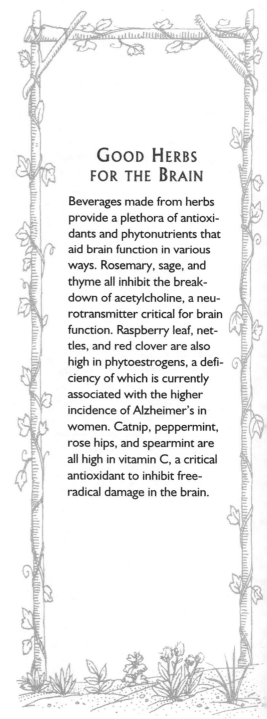

GOOD HERBS FOR THE BRAIN

Beverages made from herbs provide a plethora of antioxidants and phytonutrients that aid brain function in various ways. Rosemary, sage, and thyme all inhibit the breakdown of acetylcholine, a neurotransmitter critical for brain function. Raspberry leaf, nettles, and red clover are also high in phytoestrogens, a deficiency of which is currently associated with the higher incidence of Alzheimer's in women. Catnip, peppermint, rose hips, and spearmint are all high in vitamin C, a critical antioxidant to inhibit free-radical damage in the brain.

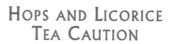

HOPS AND LICORICE TEA CAUTION

Hops are a sedative, so they should be added to teas only at night. Avoid hops if you are depressed or lacking in sexual energy. Avoid licorice if you have high blood pressure.

PRESERVE-THE-C MINT TEA

Ounce for ounce, mint has more vitamin C than oranges. Vitamin C is destroyed by heat, so make sure that the water you pour over the dried herbs is warm (less than 130 degrees Fahrenheit) and that you add the fresh sprigs after the tea has cooled. Assimilation of vitamin C is impeded by sugar consumption, so vitamin C teas are best drunk without added sweeteners. Double the amount of ingredients to make tea for two, triple for three, and so on.

LIME BLOSSOM TEA

1 teaspoon dried or 2 teaspoons fresh
1 cup of boiling water

This is an aromatic and relaxing tea that is also helpful for fevers and the flu, especially if combined with yarrow and peppermint. It induces sweating, thus helping break fevers. It is also used to reduce hardening of the arteries and high blood pressure. It can relieve vascular headaches, including migraines. It also combines well with lemon balm to ease nervous tension. Drink 1 cup three times a day.

SUSTAINING TEA

1 teaspoon dried licorice
1 teaspoon ginseng root
3 teaspoons dried borage

Boil dried licorice and ginseng root in 2 ½ cups water for 10 minutes. Pour the decoction over 3 teaspoons dried borage. Let steep for 10 minutes. Strain. Drink 1 cupful, hot or cold, three times a day. This tea will help you maintain energy and focus when under stress.

VERVAIN AND LADY'S MANTLE TEA

1 teaspoon dried vervain
1 teaspoon dried lady's mantle

Put dried vervain and dried lady's mantle into a pot. Add 1 ¼ cups boiling water. Steep for 10 minutes. Strain and sweeten to taste. Take 1 cup twice a day from day 14 of your cycle, or two weeks after your period starts. This will relieve PMS.

HOT SWEAT TEA

1 teaspoon dry sage
1 teaspoon dry motherwort

Pour 2 1/2 cups boiling water over the herbs. Sweeten with licorice (omit if you have high blood pressure). Let cool, then strain and sip throughout the day.

This tea helps to alleviate hot sweats associated with menopause. Sage is a tonic that helps alleviate stress due to change; motherwort helps to strengthen the heart. CAUTION: Do not drink sage tea continuously. Take for three weeks, then avoid for at least one week.

ROSEMARY'S MOOD SWING TEA

1 part chickweed
2 parts nettle
2 parts corn silk

1 part oatstraw
1 part uva ursi

Mix the herbs together and use 4 to 6 tablespoons per quart of water. Place cold water in a saucepan, then add the herbs and slowly bring to a simmer over low heat. Remove from heat, and keep pot covered. Infuse for 20 minutes. Strain. Drink 3 or 4 cups daily to treat PMS. It will help the body shed excess water, dispel irritability, and control mood swings that come with PMS.

REVITALIZING TEA

Wild oats
Licorice
St. John's wort

Skullcap
Borage
Wood betony

Mix equal portions of all the dried herbs above. Put 4 teaspoons of the mixture into a pot with a lid. Add 2 1/2 cups boiling water and steep for 10 minutes. Strain. Drink 3 or 4 cups a day.

REVITALIZING THE LIBIDO

Sometimes depression or anxiety makes happy sexual functioning difficult. This may be because your energy is too low, or it may be connected with a hormone imbalance. Damiana stimulates both the nervous and hormonal systems. It has constituents that convert to hormones in the body. Vervain releases tension and stress and was traditionally used as an aphrodisiac. Wild oats and ginger are both stimulating, as well. Ginger is said to fire the blood.

TONIC TEA

Wild oats   Borage
Vervain   Licorice
St. John's wort

Put ¹/₂ teaspoon each of the dried herbs into a small pot. Add boiling water. Flavor with peppermint or licorice to taste. Steep for 10 minutes and strain. Drink 3 or 4 cups (warm) each day for approximately three weeks.

This tea helps the body recover from an illness. Wild oats and St. John's wort support the nervous system, vervain promotes relaxation and digestion, and licorice and borage restore the adrenal glands. Proper recovery is vital to maintaining a healthy body. This tea will help to make sure the body receives the nutrients that it may have lost during an illness.

WINTER MOOD LIFTER

2 teaspoons St. John's wort
1 teaspoon rosemary

Combine dried St. John's wort with dried rosemary. Add 1 cup boiling water. Let steep for 10 minutes. Strain. Drink 3 times a day throughout the winter. This tea will help dispel the depression people may suffer from in the winter.

RESTORATIVE TEA

St. John's wort   Damiana
Wild oats

Mix equal parts of each of the herbs listed (dried). Put 2 teaspoons of the mixture into a pot. Add 2 ¹/₂ cups boiling water. Let steep for 10 minutes and then strain. Drink 1 cup of this tea three times a day. This will restore the health of your nervous system while having a slightly stimulating effect.

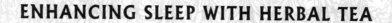

ENHANCING SLEEP WITH HERBAL TEA

Just as there are many types of people, there are also many types of insomnia. If you are having trouble sleeping, it may be a good idea to experiment with various remedies to find the one that best suits you. If you haven't been sleeping well for a long period, include a nervous system tonic to improve the long-term situation.

Drink teas made from relaxing herbs in the evenings. Lavender oil in a hot bath before bed and lavender oil on the pillow will help. You could try a hops pillow, too.

Try to allow time at the end of the day to relax and wind down. Exercise, meditation, and yoga all help with sleep difficulties. And here are some herbal remedies that may help:

Lemon balm

Chamomile

Valerian

Californian poppy

Vervain

Passionflower (use only $\frac{1}{2}$ teaspoon a day)

Hops (use $\frac{1}{2}$ teaspoon a day)

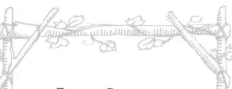

FEVER BREAKER

When you have a high temperature and suffer from a headache, make a concoction of 1 part willow bark and 5 parts water. Drink three times a day. This will help sweat the fever out and clear the head.

♥✺

HERBAL COMBINATION No. 1

These herbs are good for headache, toothache, cramps, and nerves. use them in a tea for almost any kind of pain relief.

White Willow—natural pain reliever, antiseptic properties, for cleansing and healing

Valerian—nerve tonic, headache pain reliever

Wild Lettuce—afterbirth pain reliever, general pain reliever

Capsicum—stimulant, relaxant

DIGESTIVE TEAS

Chamomile	Hops
Lemon balm	Fennel
Peppermint	Caraway
Licorice	Dill
Cramp bark	Cumin

Chamomile, hops, and lemon balm can be combined in a tea, or you can select your favorite combination. Put 1 teaspoon each of, say, lemon balm, dried chamomile flowers, and peppermint into a small teapot or mug. Add a mug of boiling water and let steep for at least 10 minutes. Strain and drink at least three times a day or after meals. This tea will relax the nervous system, encourage parasympathetic activity, and reduce spasm in the gut.

MINT TEA

1 cup water
$1\frac{1}{2}$ tablespoons fresh or $1\frac{1}{2}$ teaspoon dried peppermint or spearmint leaves
2 fresh, clean sprigs of peppermint or spearmint.

Boil 1 cup water in an open pan. Let cool five minutes. Add the dried herbs and steep until cool. Strain into a tumbler and add the mint sprigs—good additions to any tea, because the leaves can be eaten after you drink the tea for a breath-freshening finish.

GAS AND COLIC TEA

1 teaspoon fennel seeds
1 teaspoon cramp bark
1 teaspoon dried peppermint

Boil the fennel seed and cramp bark in about 1 $\frac{1}{4}$ cups of water. Add dried peppermint. Steep for 10 minutes. Strain and drink.

MORNING-AFTER TEA

1 teaspoon dried vervain
$\frac{1}{2}$ teaspoon lavender flowers

Put the herbs into a pot and add 2 $\frac{1}{2}$ cups boiling water. Cover and steep for 10 minutes. Strain and sweeten with a little honey. Sip throughout the day. This tea will help speed the body's recovery from a hangover.

SOOTHING TEA (FOR HEADACHES)

1 teaspoon dried wood betony
$\frac{1}{2}$ teaspoon dried lavender or rosemary

Put the herbs into a cup and add boiling water. Steep for 10 minutes, strain, and drink. Repeat hourly throughout the day. This tea will ease a tension headache.

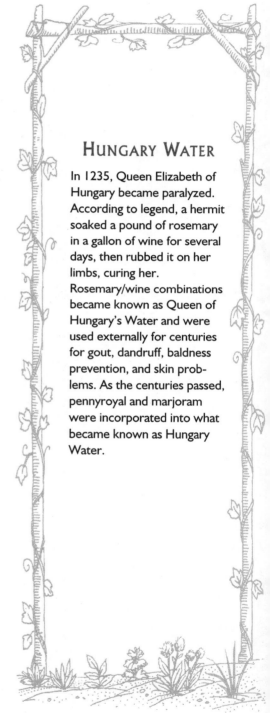

HUNGARY WATER

In 1235, Queen Elizabeth of Hungary became paralyzed. According to legend, a hermit soaked a pound of rosemary in a gallon of wine for several days, then rubbed it on her limbs, curing her. Rosemary/wine combinations became known as Queen of Hungary's Water and were used externally for centuries for gout, dandruff, baldness prevention, and skin problems. As the centuries passed, pennyroyal and marjoram were incorporated into what became known as Hungary Water.

ENERGIZING TEA

1 teaspoon dried damiana
1 teaspoon dried vervain

Put the herbs into a pot and add 2 1/2 cups of boiling water. Steep for 10 minutes. Strain and flavor with licorice, ginger, or honey. Drink 2 cups a day. This will restore energy of all kinds, including sexual energy.

SLEEPY TEA

1 teaspoon dried chamomile
1 teaspoon dried vervain
1 teaspoon dried lemon balm

Put herbs into a pot and add 2 1/2 cups boiling water. Let steep for 10 minutes. Strain and drink 1 cup after supper. Warm the rest and drink before bed. If insomnia persists, add a decoction of 1 teaspoon valerian root or 1/2 teaspoon dried hops or Californian poppy to the blend.

LICORICE TEA (FOR SORE THROATS)

1/2 teaspoon dried powdered licorice
1/2 teaspoon dried mullein or horehound
1 cup cool water

Place the water and dried herbs in a pan. Bring the mixture to a boil, remove from heat, cover, and let cool. Licorice, when combined with other herbs, will enhance their effectiveness.

POPULAR HERBAL TEAS AND THEIR USES

Alfalfa tea—aids digestion

Angelica tea—mild antispasmodic and digestive aid

Aniseed tea—decongestant for nose and sinuses

Basil and borage tea—"pick-me-up" tonic

Bilberry tea—aids circulation

Black currant tea—stimulates taste buds

Blueberry tea—pleasant before-meal tea

Borage tea—antimelancholy

Buchu tea—natural diuretic (dangerous if taken in excess)

Burdock root tea—helps sciatica and rheumatoid arthritis

Butcher's broom—good diuretic

Catnip tea—relaxant and mild depressant

Chamomile tea—calms hyperactive children, good before bedtime

Chicory tea—normalizes liver function

Cinnamon tea—clears the brain and improves thought processes

Corn silk tea—reduces pain of urinary infections

Couch grass tea—tightens and tones up the bladder sphincter, good diuretic

Dandelion tea—improves liver function and kidney function

Elder flowers tea—increases immune function

Fennel tea—good for the pancreas

Fenugreek tea—good for colds, clogged ears, and aching sinuses

Ginger tea—appetite restorer

Ginseng tea—natural tonic for a "lift"

Goldenseal root tea—internal detergent (avoid if you have high blood pressure)

Hawthorn berries tea—energizing to the elderly

Hops tea—relaxant and calming agent

Horehound tea—helps loosen heavy mucus

Jasmine tea—mild nerve sedative

Juniper berries tea—helps cystitis or bladder inflammation

Licorice tea—good laxative

Maté tea—tones muscles, especially the smooth muscles of the heart

Nettle tea—increases blood pressure (avoid if you have high blood pressure)

Orange flowers tea—sleep aid

Parsley tea—diuretic (increases flow of urine)

Peppermint tea—antigas

Raspberry tea—tightens, tones, and strengthens the uterus

Red clover tea—inner cleanser

Rosehips tea—adrenal stimulant during daytime

Sage tea—improves brain nourishment, known as the "thinker's tea"

Sarsaparilla tea—laxative, hormone balancer (should not be used on a regular basis)

Senna tea—strong laxative

Slippery elm bark tea—pain reliever

Spearmint tea—antigas

Thyme tea—sore throats and colds

Valerian tea—natural sedative

Yarrow tea—general tonic

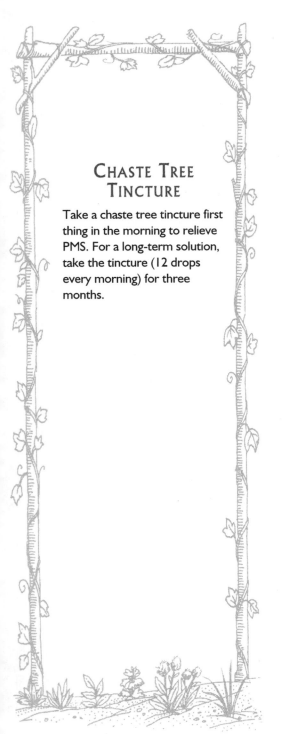

Chaste Tree Tincture

Take a chaste tree tincture first thing in the morning to relieve PMS. For a long-term solution, take the tincture (12 drops every morning) for three months.

Thyme Tea

Make a basic tea from dried thyme. Drink daily or gargle with it up to three times daily. It makes a good gargle for sore throats.

Cold Mallow Tea

2 to 3 tablespoons fresh or 2 teaspoons dried mallow
1 pint cool water

Wash the herb and break it into pieces. If the root is used, chop it. Place the herb in a jar, pour the water over it, and cover. Let it steep for 6 to 8 hours.

Take $\frac{1}{4}$ to $\frac{1}{2}$ cup three to four times daily, or more frequently if needed for stomach problems. It can be kept in the refrigerator for about five days. Or make it double strength and keep it frozen in ice cube trays; place a cube in a cup and add cold water. The tea is great for heartburn and indigestion.

The world of herbal teas is a vast and often confusing labyrinth of legend versus science; tradition versus modern technology. The recipes in this book are merely the tip of the iceberg. Almost every herb lends itself to tea-making. Your job is to find the tea(s) that best suit your needs and that are most appealing to you. There are two kinds of herbal teas: those that are used primarily as alternatives to coffee and other drinks and those that are valued for their medicinal purposes. The former are sold in most supermarkets, the herbs of which are merely used as flavoring. They are relatively weak and generally harmless, but they should not be mistaken for real herbal tea. True herbal tea is usually sold in health food stores. You can either make your own or buy tea bags. As a rule, these teas are stronger than the grocery store variety and should be used more carefully. However, before you use any herbal tea, you should learn as much as you can about the herb. If you are pregnant or have a medical condition such as high blood pressure, check with your doctor before drinking any herbal tea. Avoid stimulants such as ephedra at night or relaxing herbs such as chamomile in the morning. Some manufacturers add caffeine to their teas, so be sure to read the labels carefully. Your best bet is to buy a tea that is labeled caffeine free. If you are well informed, using herbal teas for medicinal purposes or for enjoyment is perfectly safe.

Recipes for Herbal Cough Syrups

As stated previously, a syrup is often used in treating coughs and sore throats because of its coating ability, which keeps the herbs in direct contact with the affected area. Many of us have horrible childhood memories of being forced to endure the wretched taste of a cough syrup, as if being ill weren't traumatic enough. Many of us soon realized that holding one's nose provided some small comfort when swallowing a vile-tasting syrup. The wonderful news is that we don't have to settle for those same old torturous syrups; herbal cough syrups can help!

LICORICE AND ANISE SYRUP

1 tablespoon licorice root   1 tablespoon thyme leaves
1 tablespoon crushed anise seed   1 cup honey
1 tablespoon dried bark

Gently simmer the licorice root and crushed anise seeds in 2 cups of water for 15 minutes in a covered pot. If you want to add wild cherry flavor, add 1 tablespoon dried bark and simmer with the licorice root and anise seeds. Remove from heat, add 1 tablespoon dried thyme leaves, cover, and steep until the mixture cools to room temperature. Strain, and add 1 cup of honey, warming the tea gently if necessary to completely dissolve the honey. Store in a covered glass jar in the refrigerator (it will keep for at least three months). Take 1 tablespoon as often as needed to relieve a cough.

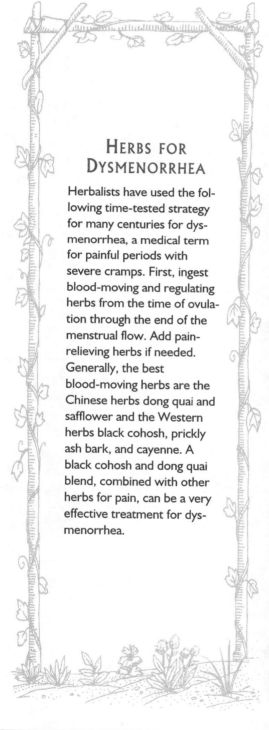

HERBS FOR DYSMENORRHEA

Herbalists have used the following time-tested strategy for many centuries for dysmenorrhea, a medical term for painful periods with severe cramps. First, ingest blood-moving and regulating herbs from the time of ovulation through the end of the menstrual flow. Add pain-relieving herbs if needed. Generally, the best blood-moving herbs are the Chinese herbs dong quai and safflower and the Western herbs black cohosh, prickly ash bark, and cayenne. A black cohosh and dong quai blend, combined with other herbs for pain, can be a very effective treatment for dysmenorrhea.

COUGH AND DECONGESTANT SYRUP

1 tablespoon dried, shaved root of apache-plume
1 tablespoon fresh or 1 teaspoon dried horehound
1 cup cool water
1 cup honey

In a saucepan, pour water over the root shavings and horehound. Bring to a boil, remove from heat, cover, and allow to sit for 20 minutes. Strain, add honey, and bring to a boil. Reduce heat and simmer for 10 minutes. Remove from heat. Pour into a jar and keep in a cool, dark place. Take 1 to 2 teaspoons for cough/congestion two to three times daily.

CRIMSON CLOVER COUGH SYRUP

1 ounce fresh or $^1/_2$ ounce dried crimson clover flowers
1 cup hot water
2 cups sugar

Put all the ingredients into a pan and bring them to a boil. Reduce heat and simmer for 10 to 15 minutes. Strain, pour the liquid into a container, and cap immediately. Store in a cool, dark place and use 1 teaspoon as needed for a cough.

SOOTHING FLAX SYRUP

$^1/_2$ ounce flax seeds
1 cup water
$^1/_4$ teaspoon lemon or lime juice
2 teaspoons honey

Put the flax seeds in a pan with water and soak until the mixture is thick. Add the juice and honey. Sip as needed for cough, sore throat, or stomach problems.

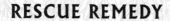

RESCUE REMEDY

Rescue Remedy can be bought as a liquid or as a cream. It is made from equal amounts of the five following essences:

- Cherry Plum—for feelings of desperation
- Rock Rose—to ease terror, fear, or panic
- Impatiens—to soothe irritability and agitation
- Clematis—to counteract the tendency to drift away from the present
- Star of Bethlehem—to address the mental and physical symptoms of shock

   When combined, these flower essences make a safe mental sanctuary in which to recover. Carry Rescue Remedy with you for all emergencies. Rescue Remedy rebalances the body after any emotional or physical trauma. It should be taken when a person is upset or in danger of going into shock. This may be after an accident, an argument, or any event that was trying on the nerves. Rescue Remedy speeds healing after surgery.
   Use Rescue Remedy cream for sunburn, cuts, bruises, and so on.

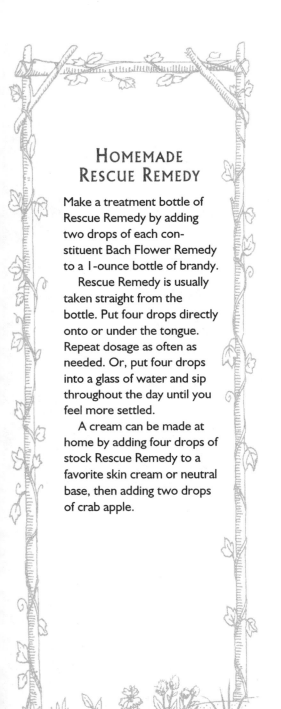

HOMEMADE RESCUE REMEDY

Make a treatment bottle of Rescue Remedy by adding two drops of each constituent Bach Flower Remedy to a 1-ounce bottle of brandy.

Rescue Remedy is usually taken straight from the bottle. Put four drops directly onto or under the tongue. Repeat dosage as often as needed. Or, put four drops into a glass of water and sip throughout the day until you feel more settled.

A cream can be made at home by adding four drops of stock Rescue Remedy to a favorite skin cream or neutral base, then adding two drops of crab apple.

HONEYSUCKLE ASTHMA AND COUGH SYRUP

1 tablespoon fresh or 1 rounded teaspoon dried honeysuckle flowers
1 tablespoon fresh or 1 rounded teaspoon dried mullein leaves
2 cups honey

Put all ingredients in a pan. Bring to a boil over low heat. Turn the heat down very low and simmer slowly for 20 minutes. Strain, then pour the syrup into a sterile bottle. Keep in a cool, dark place. Take 1 teaspoonful as needed.

HOREHOUND COUGH DROPS

2 cups sugar
1 cup water
3 tablespoons horehound leaves and stems

Boil the horehound leaves in the water for 5 minutes. Cover, then remove from the heat. Let sit for 5 minutes, then strain. Add the sugar to the liquid and bring to a boil. Cook to a hard–crack stage, then pour into a well-greased platter. Loosen the edges while the candy is cooling. Break into small pieces and use as cough drops.

MAIDENHAIR FERN SYRUP

½ cup maidenhair fern, chopped
1 teaspoon echinacea root or cone
½ cup hot water
1 cup sugar or honey

Bring the water and herbs to a boil, cover, and let the mixture steep 10 minutes. Strain, then return the liquid to the pan. Add the sugar, place over heat, and stir until the sugar is dissolved. Honey may be used instead of sugar; if this is done, add it to the strained tea and heat to boiling while stirring, then remove from heat. Place the syrup in a clean bottle or jar. A little mint or ginger can be added for taste. Take 1 teaspoon as needed for cough and congestion.

GAY-FEATHER COUGH SYRUP

½ cup fresh gay-feather roots
1 cup cold water
½ cup honey

Clean and chop the roots. Put them in a pan with the cold water, cover, and boil. Turn the heat down and simmer for 20 minutes. Strain and return the liquid to the pan and simmer for 10 more minutes. Bottle and seal the syrup and store it in a cool, dark place.

CAUTION: Pregnant women should not ingest this substance, nor should anyone taking blood thinners. It can prevent blood clotting.

It is hoped that these syrup recipes will provide you with a more pleasant source of relief than the traditional medicinal cough syrups. These herbal syrups have been in use for a long time; there has to be a good reason why they've endured so long. Try one of the recipes for yourself—it couldn't hurt.

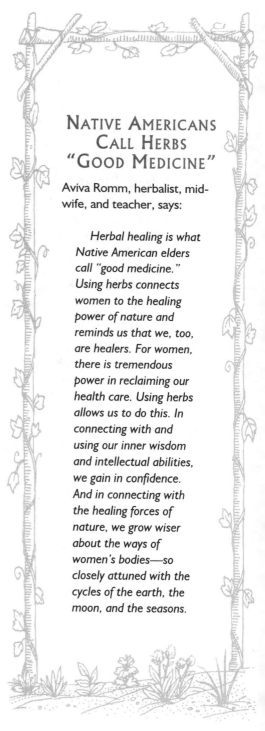

NATIVE AMERICANS CALL HERBS "GOOD MEDICINE"

Aviva Romm, herbalist, midwife, and teacher, says:

Herbal healing is what Native American elders call "good medicine." Using herbs connects women to the healing power of nature and reminds us that we, too, are healers. For women, there is tremendous power in reclaiming our health care. Using herbs allows us to do this. In connecting with and using our inner wisdom and intellectual abilities, we gain in confidence. And in connecting with the healing forces of nature, we grow wiser about the ways of women's bodies—so closely attuned with the cycles of the earth, the moon, and the seasons.

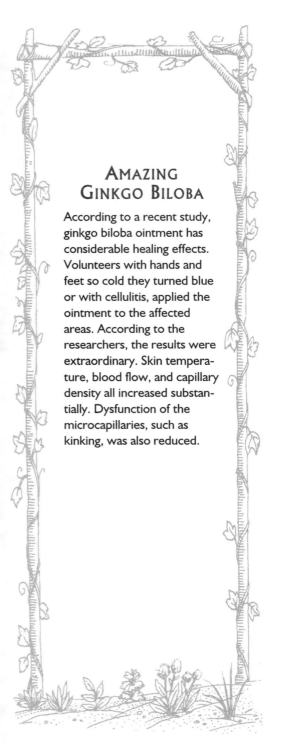

AMAZING GINKGO BILOBA

According to a recent study, ginkgo biloba ointment has considerable healing effects. Volunteers with hands and feet so cold they turned blue or with cellulitis, applied the ointment to the affected areas. According to the researchers, the results were extraordinary. Skin temperature, blood flow, and capillary density all increased substantially. Dysfunction of the microcapillaries, such as kinking, was also reduced.

Tincture Preparations

As previously stated, tinctures are highly concentrated herbal extracts that can be kept for long periods of time because the main ingredient, alcohol, is a good preservative. The final concentration of alcohol in the tincture should not be less than 30 percent. Tinctures are very useful for herbs that do not taste good or are to be taken over an extended period of time. They may also be used externally as a liniment. Some herbs, like black cohosh and chaparral, contain substances not readily extracted by water and thus should be taken as pills, capsules, or tinctures, rather than teas. Alcohol generally extracts all the important ingredients from herbs.

To make a basic tincture, combine 4 ounces of powdered or cut herb with 1 pint of alcohol, such as vodka, brandy, gin, or rum. Shake daily, allowing the herbs to steep for about two weeks. Let the herbs settle and pour off the tincture, straining out the powder through a fine cloth or filter.

Tincture dosages vary from a few drops to 2 tablespoons. This amount of alcohol is very small and should not present a problem for most people. However, people who have a history of alcoholism should avoid taking tinctures.

BLOOD-MOVING FORMULA

1 ounce black cohosh tincture
1 ounce dong quai tincture
Orange peel and licorice tinctures to taste
For pain add:
$1/2$ ounce California poppy tincture
$1/2$ ounce Jamaica dogwood tincture

Mix the tinctures and store in a dark glass bottle. Take 1 teaspoon in a little water two or three times daily between meals. Using premade tinctures makes this recipe a snap.

TEA DRINKERS ARE A LOYAL BUNCH

In *The Herbal Tea Garden*, Marietta Marshall Marcin tells us that herbal teas have been brewed for thousands of years. However, she explains, Pliny the Elder, one of the Roman statesmen who practiced advanced horticulture, advised brewing herbal teas with water and vinegar, which may very well explain why herbal teas weren't popular until they started to be brewed in water alone.

Surprisingly enough, a boost to the herbal tea market back in 1773 was otherwise known as the Boston Tea Party. Marcin tells us:

> After the Boston Tea Party, patriotic ladies banished imported tea—termed "the baneful herb" by the clergyman and educator John Andrews—from their tables and turned to domestically-grown herbal teas. They called these beverages "liberty teas." Some of their herbal combinations—made from mint, balm, rosemary, and sage—are still favorites today.

A NOTE ON CAPSULES

When making your own capsules, do not use very mild herbs that require large doses to be effective. It will not be possible to get an adequate dose this way. Also, do not mix mild-acting herbs, except those that are mucilaginous, with more potent herbs in a capsule, since the mild herbs will only dilute the potent herbs and thus will not be present in sufficient quantity to provide the desired effect.

The typical dose for herbs taken by capsule is two capsules, three times daily, though the actual dose will depend on the herb and the condition being treated. Some herbs, such as goldenseal, mandrake, poke, and lobelia, should be taken in much smaller quantities, usually by incorporating them as constituents of a larger formula. Gelatin capsules may be taken with meals but if taken between meals at least, $1/2$ cup of water or herbal tea should be used to wash them down.

TINCTURE OF BEARBERRIES

Fill a jam jar with fresh or dried bearberries. Pour vodka over the berries until they are well covered. Store in a cool place for three weeks. Shake well every few days. Strain and store in a dark bottle. The recommended dosage is 30 drops. Use for bladder and intestinal infections. Blueberries or cranberries can also be used. This tincture acts as a urinary antiseptic.

POSTMENSTRUAL FORMULA

2 ounces chasteberry seed tincture
1 ounce blue cohosh root tincture
1 ounce sarsaparilla root tincture
2 ounces milk thistle seed tincture
1 ounce partridgeberry tincture
2 ounces wild yam tincture
1 ounce valerian root tincture

Using a funnel, combine the tinctures and pour into a bottle. Take 1 teaspoon of the mixture diluted in 8 ounces of water four times a day, from the time your period ends until ovulation. This will stimulate tissue health, balance hormones, enhance liver function, shrink benign growths, and ease pain.

The recipes in this section, are merely a starting point. You can make your own remedies to suit your own needs. The ritual of making your own medicines is powerful medicine in itself. When you make a remedy, you're affirming that you want to get better, and you're putting positive energy into the healing process. Besides, making tinctures and other herbal remedies is as easy as making soup—and it can be just as beneficial.

Creams, Ointments, and Salves

Ointments and salves are preparations that can be applied to the skin and remain in place due to their thick consistency. A salve can be made by first preparing an herbal oil, heating it, and then adding melted beeswax to obtain the desired consistency (about 1 ½ ounces per pint of oil). The quickest method is to allow about 2 hours for roots and barks to extract in oil heated to just below boiling point. Keep the pot covered. Next, add leaves and flowers and continue to cook gently for another hour. Then add the melted wax and stir well. Or mix one part of the powdered herbs into four parts of hot lard or other fat that is hard at room temperature. With either method, add a small amount of gum benzoin or tincture of benzoin to the salve to help preserve it (1 teaspoon of the tincture per quart of salve). Salves and ointments are generally used for their antiseptic properties in cases of cuts and scrapes.

Acne Treatment

2 ounces chopped bee balm
4 ounces alcohol

Wash the bee balm, dry it, and place it in a jar. Add the alcohol, making sure the herb is totally submerged. Keep in a dark place, shaking the jar frequently. After 14 days, strain into a bottle, cap tightly, and store in a dark place. After washing and drying the skin, apply the solution to pimples as needed.

Cinquefoil Tea for Topical Use

1 well-rounded teaspoon of cinquefoil root
1 ½ cups cool water

Bring the water and root to a boil. Simmer, covered, for 20 minutes. Allow to cool. This tea is great as a topical treatment for mouth ulcers, as a gargle for sore throats, and to get rid of warts.

COPPER CANYON MARIGOLD FIRST-AID SALVE

1 cup chopped copper canyon marigold or $\frac{1}{2}$ cup of the
dried herb (use any part except the root)
$\frac{1}{2}$ cup vegetable shortening

Melt the shortening in a pan. Stir in the herb. Set the pan into another pan of boiling water (a double boiler). Leave uncovered for 1 hour, stirring occasionally. With fresh herbs, the ointment will keep only for a short time. With dried herbs, it will keep well.

DOCK LEAVES FOR STINGING NETTLE

Dock has long been used as a treatment for the skin irritation caused by stinging nettle. The mashed dock leaves are rubbed directly on the affected part. This relieves the sting of nettle.

GOLDENROD SALVE FOR STINGS

1 cup goldenrod flowers, chopped
$\frac{1}{2}$ cup shortening

In a double boiler, heat the shortening until it melts. Stir in the chopped flowers and cook in this manner for 45 minutes. Pour into a container to cool. The salve will keep better if it is stored in the refrigerator.

ALOE GEL

Aloe vera leaves

Wash the aloe leaves. Cut into 2-inch lengths. Slice each piece in half to expose the largest amount of gel. Wrap each piece in plastic wrap and date. To use, remove plastic and apply the gel side of the leaf to the skin. Smear over the affected area, or hold in place with a bandage. Apply to burns, sunburn, ringworm, infected cuts, acne, shingles, eczema, wrinkles, and areas of dry, itchy skin.

MARSH MALLOW PASTE

Marsh mallow root powder

Take enough marsh mallow root powder to cover the affected area and add cold water to make a stiff paste. Apply thickly and allow to dry. Wash off and replace the paste every 2 or 3 hours. This treatment is especially good for insect bites and stings.

POPPY SEED SALVE

6 tablespoons crushed prickly poppy seeds
6 tablespoons petroleum jelly or lard

Put the seeds and petroleum jelly or lard in a small pan. Put the pan into a larger pan that has water in it (or use a double boiler). Boil the water. Stir the mixture until it melts. Turn the heat to low and leave the pan on the heat for 1 to 2 hours. Strain the mixture into jars and seal.

This salve is good for minor burns, hemorrhoids, itching, ulcers, scrapes, and other painful skin conditions. Do not use it for serious burns.

SUPER SUNBURN SALVE

Aloe vera (liquid)
For sunburns, combine liquid aloe vera with half as much liquid vitamin E and a few drops of lavender oil in a spray bottle. Lightly mist over sensitive skin and watch the color and heat fade!

These herbal alternatives may prove to be well worth the effort to keep around the house, especially if you have children. Someone always has a scrape or bruise to be tended. What better way is there to show your love than to make the medicine yourself?

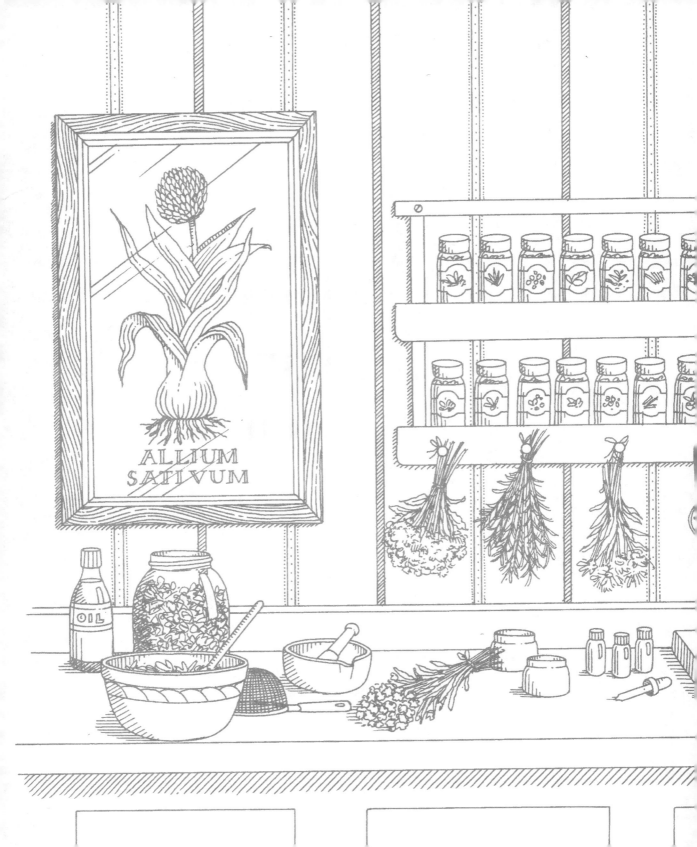

ALLIUM
SATIVUM

OIL

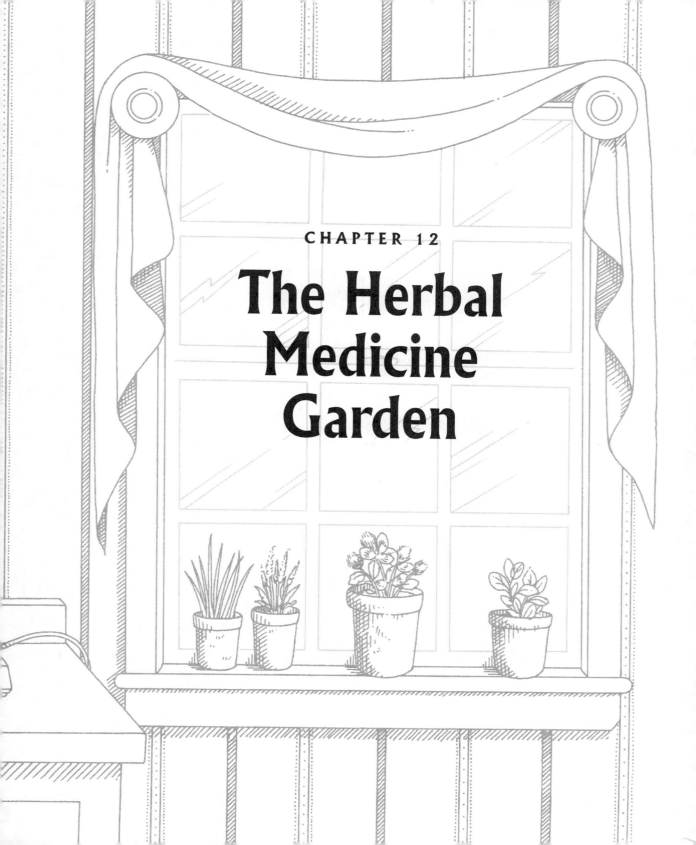

CHAPTER 12

The Herbal Medicine Garden

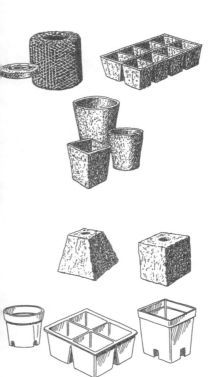

G rowing your own medicinal herbs may seem a daunting idea to those who consider themselves nongardeners or who claim they don't have a "green thumb." But the good news is that the herbs themselves are all thumbs—green ones, that is. Herbs will grow just about anywhere and under a wide variety of conditions. They require minimal care and are quite willing to thrive in tiny spaces, and almost all of them can be grown successfully in pots on a windowsill or in window boxes.

If you have a little garden space outside, that's a bonus; herbs take up little space and serve as protectors for other plants, repelling insects and plant diseases. Thus, herbs protect *human* health and are guardians of the garden as well!

Depending on your temperament, time, and space available, you can start small—with a pot or a few pots on a sunny windowsill—and gradually expand as your means allow. Herbs are not expensive, either as already started plants or as seeds, and they are extremely rewarding. Many healing herbs are also useful as culinary herbs, such as rosemary, sage, thyme, and lemon balm.

Many herbs grow wild, of course, and can easily be transplanted into a pot or a garden space. You can forage along roadsides (where permitted) and bring home whole uprooted plants, always being sure to handle them with care and never taking more than one or two.

Another wonderful thing about growing your own herbs is that a little goes a long way. Fresh herbs are very potent, and just a few sprigs of rosemary or parsley, for example, can make a tea or an infusion. And even if you don't have a sunny windowsill, grow lights are available so that the indoor gardener without benefit of direct sun can still have a plot of herbs available.

Ideally, herbs prefer a lot of sun—eight hours a day if possible in northern climates. In the southern and western states where the sun can burn ferociously all day long, they need to be shaded from the heat of the day—as even sun-loving herbs can suffer sunburn. When buying herbs for a garden, be sure to take into consideration the planting zone in which you live.

In addition to being beneficial for your health, herbs are attractive as well. Most herbs like well-drained soil, and if you are going to put them in pots, first line the pot with a layer of small gravel or pebbles (sometimes called "pea gravel") to provide good drainage. Herbs in pots need frequent watering, especially if they are outside in the full sun. However, do not water them so much that they become soggy, which can cause root rot.

A half-size galvanized tub with holes punched in the bottom (using a Phillips screwdriver and a hammer) makes an ideal container for a collection of herb plants. It's big enough to contain several plants and deep enough to give the roots plenty of room to expand their range. Also, used outside, it will require less frequent watering. Again, be sure to use a layer of gravel in the bottom.

Another way to make sure your soil is herb friendly in terms of drainage is to use a soil conditioner such as Perma Till or Profile (available at local garden shops or nurseries) and to mix sand in with the potting soil. Leaf mold is another good addition for better drainage. However, there are also specially prepared potting soils already mixed with peat moss, vermiculite, sand, and special moisturizing pellets, available at garden stores and nurseries. So even the most time-pressed person who wants to grow herbs has little excuse for not making the effort.

Growing herbs is a wonderful way to get back to the simple basics of life. Herbs are especially rewarding as "house pets," as their needs are minimal—you don't have to walk them or clean litter pans! Just a little loving care will give you great pleasure, increase your health, and make you feel closer to Nature.

Many herbs can be grown successfully from seeds, especially members of the carrot family, such as dill, fennel, chervil, coriander (cilantro), and parsley. However, these herbs don't like being transplanted, so they should be seeded directly into the container (or ground space) in which they are going to grow. For growing other herbs from seed for transplanting, garden stores sell special seed-starter soil mixes; when seedlings are about 3 inches high, they can be transplanted to larger pots. Remember that both mineral

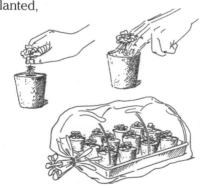

NURTURE AN HERB, NURTURE YOURSELF

In The *Woman's Book of Healing Herbs,* Sharol Tilgner, N.D., naturopathic doctor and herbalist, talks about the importance of herbs in women's lives:

From planting a seed to making and using an herbal medicine, herbalism can enrich women's lives on multiple levels. Growing an herb creates an intimacy with nature. Nurturing that herb can teach women how to nurture themselves. Learning to make teas, poultices, herbal baths, and other herbal preparations for personal health care can be self-empowering. And the process of making these medicinal preparations becomes a welcome ritual in today's hectic society.

GROWING CHINESE HERBS

Yes, you can raise these exotic plants in your own home! Now, Oregon Exotics Nursery carries a wide variety of medicinal plants from all corners of the globe. From China, they offer a large variety, including chaste-berry and astragalus. For a catalog, send a check or money order to Oregon Exotics, 1065 Messinger Road, Grants Pass, Oregon 97527.

WEEDS YOU CAN USE!

- **Chicory** is used to relieve indigestion.
- **Dandelion** is used as a diuretic and laxative.
- **Plantain** is used for treating minor wounds.
- **Saw palmetto** is used to treat benign prostate enlargement.
- **St. John's wort** is used to treat mild to moderate depression.
- **Stinging nettle** is used to treat benign prostate enlargement.
- **Yarrow** is used to ease muscle spasms.

and enzyme concentrations in the soil nourish the plant, so get expert advice at your plant store about different soil compositions.

When planting outside in the garden, herbs are usually best when planted in the fall, before the ground freezes, so that they can establish a firm root system before winter sets in. However, in extremely cold climates, herbs should be planted in early spring as soon as the ground can be worked. To get an early start, seedlings can be started indoors for later transplanting to the garden.

Annual herbs usually reseed themselves—such plants as borage, lemon balm, feverfew, chives, pennyroyal, and sweet violet spring up again every year. The woody perennials like lavender, rosemary, and thyme don't produce their own offspring, but once they become established plants, they tend to grow into large plants. Rosemary especially is prone to lush growth and, when given a larger pot from time to time, will eventually produce a bushy plant.

Some plants, like mint and tarragon, can only be propagated from cuttings or divisions. The best thing to do is to purchase these from a good nursery. Be careful with mints, however, especially in the garden, as they can take over in record time. A good idea for mint is to plant it in a large pot sunk into the ground to keep it contained.

Fortunately, most herbs do well in containers, so if you don't have much space—or an outside garden (if you live in an apartment in a city)—you can grow all your herbs in pots. Personally, I prefer growing herbs in pots and other containers because I can move them around to either catch more sun or to protect them from excessive sun, and I can use them inside as decorative and aromatic plants as well. To accommodate my inside herb garden, I bought a baker's rack (one of those wire multishelved stands that originally were used by bakers to cool pies and cakes) and set it in front of a window that faces due east and gets full sun from dawn until midday. When the sunlight is wan, the herbs are cozy warm inside and flourish under grow lights.

When you discover how easy it is to grow herbs, you will likely collect them avidly and tuck them into odd places about your yard or house.

WHERE TO PURCHASE HERBS

Most nurseries carry quite a few herbs both in seed packets and as robust seedlings ready to transplant into a pot. Look for a good nursery in your area and talk to the people who run it—ask to see the manager or horticulturist on staff and don't hesitate to get as much information as you can about your particular needs—including soil conditions, availability of sun, containers, potting soil mixes, and so on.

You can also avail yourself of the specialty catalogs. Most of these companies also have trained staff available to answer your questions and give advice, and they are happy to do so. Here are a few sources:

Companion Plants
7247 North Coolville Ridge Road
Athens, Ohio 45701

They have over a hundred varieties of seeds and three hundred varieties of plants.

The Rosemary House
120 South Market Street
Mechanicsburg, Pennsylvania 17055

They carry a hundred varieties of plants and two hundred varieties of seeds.

Taylor's Herb Gardens, Inc.
1535 Lone Oak Road
Vista, California 92084

They stock a variety of plants.

Abundant Life Seed Foundation
Post Office Box 772
Port Townsend, Washington 98368

Directories of Herbal Sources

The Herb Gardener's Mail-Order Source Book by Elayne Moos
Woodsong Graphics
Post Office Box 238
New Hope, Pennsylvania 18938

This book contains one hundred and thirty listings of herbal sources.

North Wind Farm Directory by Paula Oliver
Route 2, Post Office Box 246
Shevlin, Minnesota 56676

This book contains eight hundred listings and is updated annually.

The International Herb Growers and Marketers Association
Post Office Box 281
Silver Spring, Pennsylvania 17575

GARLIC

If you grow only one herb, make it garlic. "Garlic is one of the most powerful medicinal plants there is," says David Winston, a professional member of the AHG and founder of Herbalist and Alchemist. Used as medicine for millennia, garlic has repeatedly shown an ability to kill viruses and bacteria. Researchers attribute its healing powers to allicin, a compound released when the bulb is cut or crushed. According to Winston, "It's the oil that possesses the antibacterial activity." Winston advises consuming at least I teaspoon of crushed garlic a day (that's one large clove)—easy enough to do as an addition to salad or practically any cooked dish. And, if you prefer to take a supplement, choose a gelcap variety that contains pure garlic oil rather than an "odorless" tablet.

Harvesting and Storing Herbs

You can harvest the leaves of medicinal herbs—or those you want to use for culinary use as well—at any time during the growing season. Be sure they are green and fresh and avoid harvesting any that may have turned brown or greyish. Color is important; it is an indication that the plant may have been attacked by bugs or disease. Discard any such plants and remove them from contact with healthy plants. If harvesting herbal flowers, cut them *before* they have come into full bloom.

Drying and Storing Seeds

If you are collecting seeds, be sure the seed pod is completely ripe. It should snap off easily in your hand. When you are collecting seeds, use small paper bags and mark them so that you will know later which seeds are in which bags. Seeds must be dried promptly so that small amounts of undetected moisture don't lead to rotting while the seed is in storage. To complete the drying process, put small quantities of seed in labeled paper bags and place the bags in a warm spot with good air circulation where they will not be subject to moisture. Shake the bags daily to stir the seeds around and help the drying process. Larger quantities of seed can be spread in a single layer over wax or parchment paper (available at kitchen supply stores) and put on racks (the kind used for cooling cookies), or they can be laid in a shallow cardboard box (a box lid is a good container for this). If the weather is humid, you can hasten drying and prevent rot by placing the seeds a few inches from a light bulb (an art lamp or gooseneck lamp is a good choice). Don't try to dry seeds in an oven, as heat can damage them.

Drying and Storing Herbs

Healing herbs, whether used singly or in combination, almost always are made from the dried plant material, whether it is leaves, stems, roots, flowers, or other plant parts. The traditional method of drying herbs is fairly simple. Gather the herbs in bunches, tie, and hang in a warm, dry spot (perhaps in a barn or garage) until they are easily crumbled between your fingers,

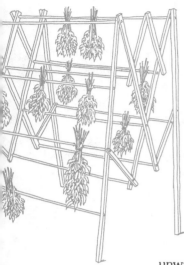

then store. Dried herbs should be stored in airtight, clean, screw-top jars (of the Mason preserving type) and should be replaced yearly, as their potency wanes with time. They should also be kept away from light and heat.

You can store your herbs in cut and dried form, or you can make them into powder (especially if you want to fill your own capsules) by using a mortar and pestle. Just make sure the mortar and pestle is clean and dry, and that you wash and dry them thoroughly after each use for each different herb so as not to make unwanted combinations. If a mortar and pestle seem like too much work (actually it's quite easy, but to each his own method), you can grind herbs in a small electric herb grinder made for the purpose (generally available through kitchen supply catalogs like Williams Sonoma), or use a coffee grinder. However, if you use a coffee grinder, reserve it for grinding herbs and don't also use it for grinding coffee.

Moisture is an enemy of dried herbs. To combat this, you can use the little antimoisture packets that often come packed with vitamins, or you can stuff the top of the container with cotton wadding to prevent moisture from creeping in. Check them occasionally for any hint of mold or insect infestation (though usually insects are repelled by strongly aromatic herbs). After using a portion from a container, make sure you close it tightly.

Tinctures made from the dried herbs should be kept in tightly closed dark glass bottles, in a cool, dry place, in which they will last for two or three years.

Storing Fresh Herbs

There's nothing more tantalizing than the aroma and flavor of freshly cut herbs from the garden. And undoubtedly the fresh plant is more nutritious and potent than its dried form. Unfortunately, fresh herbs are hard to keep for more than one or two days (rose-

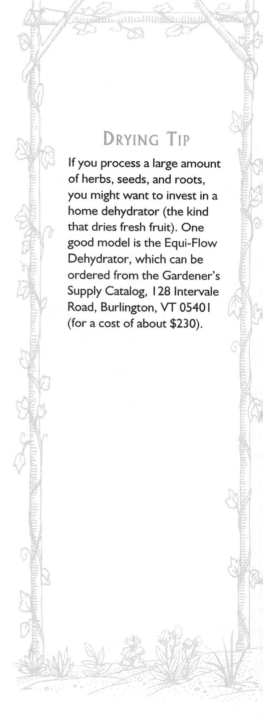

DRYING TIP

If you process a large amount of herbs, seeds, and roots, you might want to invest in a home dehydrator (the kind that dries fresh fruit). One good model is the Equi-Flow Dehydrator, which can be ordered from the Gardener's Supply Catalog, 128 Intervale Road, Burlington, VT 05401 (for a cost of about $230).

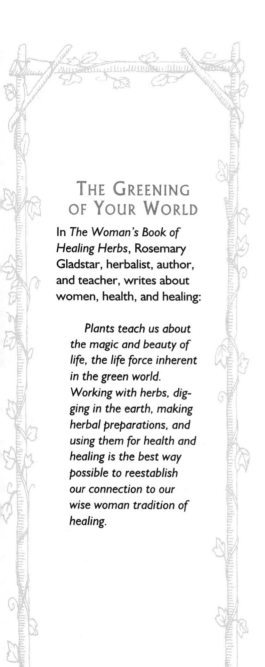

THE GREENING OF YOUR WORLD

In *The Woman's Book of Healing Herbs*, Rosemary Gladstar, herbalist, author, and teacher, writes about women, health, and healing:

Plants teach us about the magic and beauty of life, the life force inherent in the green world. Working with herbs, digging in the earth, making herbal preparations, and using them for health and healing is the best way possible to reestablish our connection to our wise woman tradition of healing.

mary is a notable exception and will keep in the refrigerator in a glass jar tightly sealed for one or two weeks). So, what can you do? For one thing, whether you get your fresh herbs from your garden or from the supermarket, refrigerate them at once. Glass jars are better than plastic bags because they allow less moisture (which causes rot) to enter and wet leaves quickly spoil. *Do not wash herbs before storing them in the refrigerator.* One way to keep fresh herbs longer is to put the stems in a jar or glass with just an inch or so of water in the bottom and cover with a plastic bag (this acts like a little greenhouse and is a good way of preserving lettuce and green onions, too).

The best method for storing fresh herbs (that you don't want to dry) is to wash them, blot dry with paper towels (or use a salad spinner), chop them (a food processor is excellent for this) and put them into ice cube trays half-filled with water, and freeze them.

You will then have the fresh herb available whenever you want, either for making a medicinal herbal tea (or infusion), or for flavoring food. Either use a spoon or shake some dried herb into the palm of your hand before adding to the liquid. (When using herbs for cooking or making teas, *never* shake the herb out of the bottle into steaming liquid; the rising steam could get into the bottle and turn the contents moldy. It's also a good idea to rub the herb between your palms to release the volatile oils before dropping it into the water.

Another freezing method, though more cumbersome than the ice cube tray method, works well if you have a freezer with plenty of space. Simply spread the washed and dried chopped herbs on cookie sheets in a single layer and freeze until hard; this will take one or two hours, depending on the freezer's temperature. Then, break the rigid sheets of herbs into pieces, place them in small freezer bags (pressing out all the air before sealing the bag) and store them in the freezer.

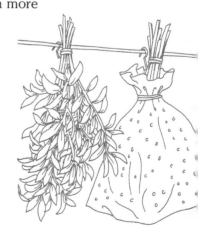

HERBAL GARDENS IN COLONIAL AMERICA

Our colonial ancestors set great store by herbs and used them as much as they had in "the old country." If the farm or cottage didn't have a "proper" herb garden, all gardens had at least a corner where herbs were grown. Many of these herb gardens of the old colonial mansions were planted in the formal designs of the English garden, and we can still see these in colonial Williamsburg, Pennsylvania. The Native Americans used "weeds" that grew in the fields and forests for herb teas and medicines, and the colonial housewife often consulted her "squaw" neighbor for advice on which plants were safe to use and for what.

Today, herbs have become once more a part of our daily lives, whether we purchase them in a health food store or take the trouble to grow them ourselves. They are easy to cultivate, and few gardening efforts are less troublesome or more rewarding than growing herbs of one's own. What better way to reconnect to Nature and our own natures?

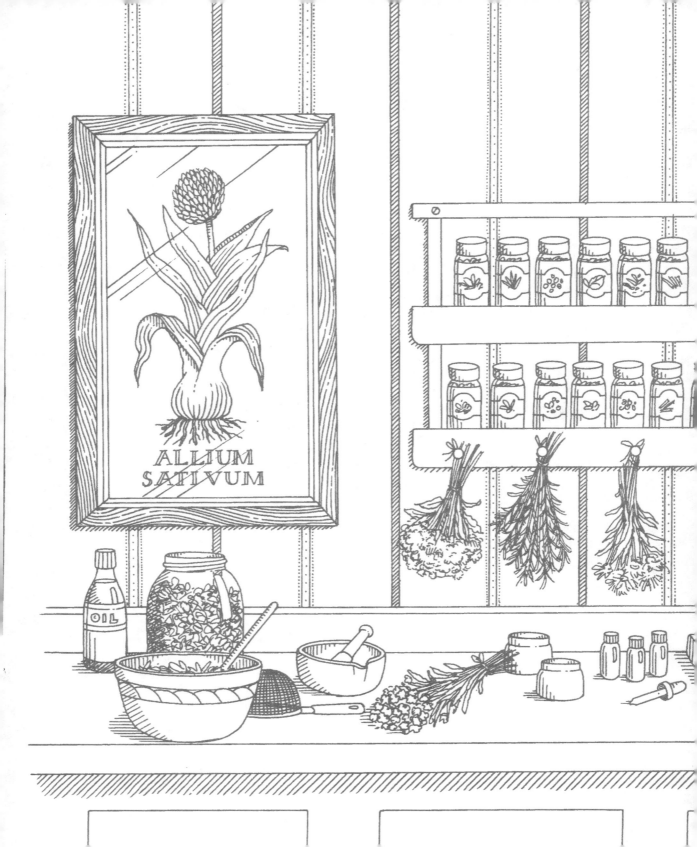

ALLIUM
SATIVUM

OIL

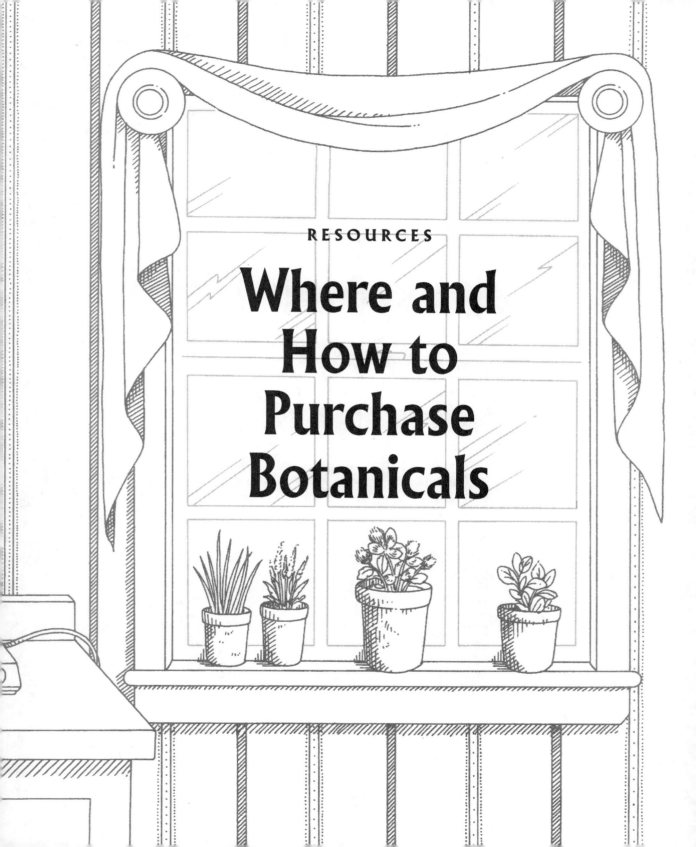

RESOURCES

Where and How to Purchase Botanicals

H undreds of herbs are regularly available today in many forms and at all quality levels. Improved storage and worldwide communications allow us to work with herbs from different countries and different harvests at the same time.

The most commonly used herbs can be obtained through a good herb or health food store. More rare or exotic herbs may have to be obtained from specialty sources (if they are available); not all are sold in the United States. Check your area for a good health food store or a herb specialty shop.

If you cannot find the herbal products or materials you want, it is possible to obtain many through mail order. The following list contains the names, addresses, and phone numbers of suppliers of high-quality herbs. Some offer catalogs; some do not. Some will provide consultation; others do not. Some are retailers who sell in small quantities; others are wholesalers who sell herbs by the pound.

The best way to find out about any particular supplier is to write or telephone and ask about their products and whether a catalog is available. As herbalists and herb sellers tend to be dedicated people, you can expect a polite response to your inquiry. And you can trust in the quality of their herbal products. Usually, they have herbal knowledge and are willing to share it with the customer. However, it is still important for you to learn what healing herbs smell, feel, and taste like. Most herbs are identified accurately, but adulteration is still possible—particularly among such costly herbs as saffron, ginseng, goldenseal, and echinacea. When buying herbs in bulk, test them before use.

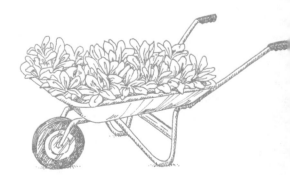

Suppliers

Acta Health Products
1979 East Locust Street
Pasadena, California 91107

Aloe Life International
4822 Santa Monica Avenue,
#231
San Diego, California 92107
800-414-2563

American Health and Herbs
Post Office Box 940
Philomath, Oregon 97370
800-345-4152

Beehive Botanicals
Route 8, Post Office Box 8257
Hayward, Wisconsin 54843
800-233-4483

Bio-Botanica, Inc.
75 Commerce Drive
Hauppauge, New York 11788
516-231-5522

Body Ecology
295 King Road
Atlanta, Georgia 30342
800-478-3842

Burt's Bees
Post Office Box 90157
Raleigh, North Carolina
  27675-0157
919-510-8720

Desert Essence
9510 Vassar Avenue, Unit A
Chatsworth, California 91311
800-645-5768

Diamond Herpanacine Assocs.
Post Office Box 544
Ambler, Pennsylvania 19002
215-542-2981

Earthrise Company
Post Office Box 1196
San Rafael, California 94915
415-485-0521

Ecco Bella Botanicals, Inc.
1133 Route 23 S.
Wayne, New Jersey 07470
201-696-7766

Eclectic Institute
11231 S. E. Market Street
Portland, Oregon 97216
800-332-HERB

Educated Beauty Inc.
77 Digital Drive
Novato, California 94949
888-323-8423

Elizabeth Van Buren, Inc.
303 Potrero Street, #33
Santa Cruz, California 95060
800-710-7759

Excel
3280 West Hacienda
Las Vegas, Nevada 89041
702-795-7464

Four Seasons Herb Co.
17 Buccaneer Street
Marina Del Rey, California
90292

Golden Gate Herbs, Inc.
Post Office Box 810
Occidental, California 95465

Haussmann's Pharmacy
534-535 W. Girard Avenue
Philadelphia, Pennsylvania
19123

The Herb and Spice
Collection
Post Office Box 118
Norway, Iowa 52318

Herbal Products/Development
Post Office Box 1084
Aptos, California 95001
408-688-8706

HerbPharm's Whole Herb
  Catalog
Post Office Box 116
Williams, Oregon 97544

Herbs for Kids
151 Evergreen Drive, Suite D
Bozeman, Montana 59715
406-587-0180

In Life Energy Systems
Red Marine Algae
107 California Avenue
Mill Valley, California 94941
415-389-1738

Indiana Botanic Gardens, Inc.
Post Office Box 5
Hammond, Indiana 46325

Innovative Natural Products
640 Alpine Way
Escondido, California 92029
800-266-4447

Jarrow Formulas
1824 South Robertson
Boulevard
Los Angeles, California 90035
310-204-6936

Kwan Yin Chinese Herb Co.,
Inc.
Post Office Box 18617
Spokane, Washington 99208

Live Food Products, Inc.
Post Office Box 7
Santa Barbara, California 93102
800-446-1990

Maine Coast Sea Vegetables
RR1, Post Office Box 78
Franklin, Maine 04634
207-565-2907

McZand Herbal Inc.
Post Office Box 5312
Santa Monica, California 90409
310-822-0500

Mendocino Sea Vegetable Co.
Post Office Box 1265
Mendocino, California 95460
707-937-2050

Motherlove Herbal Co.
Post Office Box 101
Laporte, Colorado 80535
970-493-2892

Nature's Alchemy/Lotus Brands,
Inc.
Post Office Box 325
Twin Lakes, Wisconsin 53181
800-824-6396

Nature's Herb Co.
281 Ellis Street
San Francisco, California 94102

Nature's Herbs
1010 46th Street
Emeryville, California 04608

Nature's Herbs
113 North Industrial Park Drive
Orem, Utah 84057
801-225-4443

Nature's Way
Post Office Box 4000
Springville, Utah 84883
800-9-NATURE

New Chapter
99 Main Street
Brattleboro, Vermont 05301
800-543-7279

Nutricology
Post Office Box 489
400 Preda Street
San Leandro, California
94577-0489
800-545-9960

Oshadhi Essential Oils
32422 Alipaz, Suite C
San Juan Capistrano,
California 92675
800-933-1008

Phyto-Pharmica
Post Office Box 1348
Green Bay, Wisconsin 54305

Premier Labs
27475 Ynez Road, Suite 305
Temecula, California 92591
909-699-8801

Prevail Corp.
2204-8 N.W. Birdsdale
Gresham, Oregon 97030
800-248-0885

Solaray
Ogden, Utah 84663

Source Naturals
19 Janis Way
Scotts Valley, California 95066
800-815-2333

Starwest Botanicals
11253 Trade Center Drive
Rancho Cordova, California
95742
800-800-4372

Threshold
23 Janesway
Scotts Valley, California 95066
408-438-1144

Trout Lake Farm Co.
149 Little Mountain Road
Trout Lake, Washington 98650
800-395-6093

Vagosang Skin Care System
55 West Sunset Way
Issaquah, Washington 98027
206-557-4605

Waddell Creek Organic Bee
Farm
654 Swanton Road
Davenport, California 95017

Wakunaga of America Co., Ltd.
23501 Madero
Mission Viejo, California
   92691-2764
714-855-2776

Yerba Prima
Post Office Box 5009
Berkeley, California 94705
415-632-7477

Y.S. Royal Jelly and
   Organic Bee Farm
Route 1, Post Office Box 91-A
Sheridan, Illinois 60551
800-654-4593

IN CANADA:
BIO-FORCE
4001 Cote Verth
Montreal, Quebec H4R1R5

Flora Distributors Ltd.
7400 Fraser Park Drive
Burnaby, British Columbia
V5J5B9
604-438-1133

The Herb Works
Post Office Box 450
Fergus, Ontario N1M1N8
519-824-4280
Nu-Life Nutrition, Ltd.
871 Beatty Street
Vancouver, British Columbia

QUEST
1781 W. 75th Avenue
Vancouver, British Columbia
V6P6P2
604-261-0611

Swiss Herbal Remedies
181 Don Park Road
Markham, Ontario L3R1C2
416-475-6345

Trophic Canada Ltd.
260 Okanagan Avenue East
Penticton, British Columbia
V2A357
604-492-8820

VITA Health
150 Beghin Avenue
Winnipeg, Manitoba R2J3W2
204-661-8386

IN BRITAIN:
Baldwins
171-173 Walworth Road
London SE17
071-703-5550

Brome and Schimmer Ltd
5 Great Bridge Road Estate
Romsey
Hampshire SO5 0HR
0794-515-595

Neal's Yard Apothecary
2 Neal's Yard
Covent Garden
London WC2
071-379-7222

Phytoproducts
Tidebrook Manor Farm
Wadhurst
Sussex TN5 6PD

Pierce A. Arnold and Son
Pollard Road
Morden
Surrey SM4 6EG
081-647-5330

Potters Ltd.
Leyland Mill Lane
Widan
Lancashire WN1 2SB
0942-34761

SHOP ON-LINE

Now you don't even have to change out of your pajamas to stock up on your favorite natural foods. Wild Oats Markets, a natural foods retailer, has just opened a store on-line. Stop in at *http://shopwildoats.com*, and browse the selection of more than a thousand organic grocery items—vitamins, minerals, and herbal supplements, natural toiletries, and gourmet gift baskets—it's all there, at the click of a mouse. The site includes pictures, descriptions, ingredients, and even nutritional profiles. Place your order and have all the products you can't find in nowhere-ville, USA, shipped directly to your door. There's no waiting in line, no screaming children, and no crazed shoppers trying to drive over you with their carts—just you, your computer, and maybe a cup of tea while you shop.

Index